Caribbean Youth Development

Issues and Policy Directions

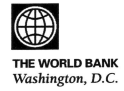

THE WORLD BANK
Washington, D.C.

CONTENTS

LIST OF TABLES

LIST OF FIGURES

LIST OF BOXES

FOREWORD

Young people are the custodians of our society and the trustees of prosperity for future generations. Nowhere is this more apparent than the Caribbean region, where two-thirds of the population is under the age of 30. This "youthful profile" of the Caribbean nations presents both opportunities and challenges in the years ahead as the important role that young people play in national and regional development becomes increasingly apparent.

Experience has taught us that young people can play an important role in national development if provided the right tools, the learning and empowerment to employ those tools and a supportive environment in which to use them. Young people can and should lead the way in economic growth and poverty reduction. By the same token, however, that same energy and vitality, if left unharnessed or if marginalized can have a dramatic negative effect on social and economic stability.

This study, undertaken at the request of our clients, could not be more timely or relevant for our work in the Caribbean Region, where we have witnessed a worrying upward trend in youth-associated issues of drug trafficking, HIV/AIDs infection, adolescent pregnancies, and other risky behavior. Set against a backdrop of regional and international instability, the urgency of grappling with this vital component of society has pushed the Bank to explore innovative measures to address and include youth as an integral part of our work.

The study is the first work of its kind to present quantitative evidence that investing in youth is an economically sound approach for Governments to take. The authors recognize, however, that the area of youth and development is an often complex and uncomfortable one to address, as many of the possible solutions entail behavioral changes that challenge long-established and accepted norms. This study will, we hope, encourage and stimulate the dialogue on youth in the region and assist those working in this critical area—Governments, Youth Organizations, NGOs, the donor community and young people themselves—in framing workplans for breaking the cycle of inter-generational poverty.

Orsalia Kalantzopoulos
Director, Caribbean Country Management Unit
Latin America and the Caribbean Region

PREFACE

This report examines youth development in the Caribbean today. Organized into seven chapters, the report provides an overview of the risks Caribbean youth are facing, evidence of the protective and risk factors underlying the problems youth are facing, an estimation of costs of risky youth behaviors, and an overview of the policy framework and the types of programs in place that target youth. The report responds directly to a request by the Caribbean Group for Cooperation and Economic Development at its 2000 consultative meeting for the World Bank to analyze the situation of Caribbean youth. It also provides an important input into the Bank's strategic social agenda for the Caribbean.

The report also follows on other World Bank economic and sector work prepared in the Caribbean, including "A Review of Gender Issues in the Dominican Republic, Haiti and Jamaica" report (21866-LAC, May 2001), the "Dominican Republic Poverty Assessment" (21306-DR, January 16, 2001); the "Trinidad and Tobago Youth and Social Development" report (20088-TR, June 2000), the "HIV/AIDS in the Caribbean: Issues and Options" report (20491-LAC, June 2000); and the "Violence and Urban Poverty in Jamaica: Breaking the Cycle" report (15895-JM, January 1997).

The report was based on a multistage process, which involved carrying out consultations with government and civil society representatives in Barbados and St. Lucia in March 2002, carrying out focus groups and semi-structured interviews with key experts in St. Lucia and the Dominican Republic in February and March 2002, conducting an authors' meeting in the Dominican Republic in April 2002 to identify key lessons and policy recommendations, and carrying out consultations on key findings and main messages with government and civil society stakeholders in the Dominican Republic and Jamaica (including youth groups in both countries) in April and May 2002, respectively, and with youth representatives and government officials from the English-speaking Caribbean at the Commonwealth Youth Programme's (CYP) regional forum in the British Virgin Islands in October 2002.

Wendy Cunningham and Maria Correia (World Bank) wrote this report based on background papers prepared by Robert Blum, Lincoln Williams, David Luther, Julia Hasbún, and Arlette St. Ville (consultants) and Wendy Cunningham and Enrique Hennings (World Bank); expert advice from Patrice Lafleur and Armstrong Alexis (CYP); and invaluable peer review from Gary Barker (consultant). The country director is Orsalia Kalantzopoulos, the lead economist is Antonella Bassani, the sector director is Ernesto May, the chief economist is Guillermo Perry, and the vice president is David de Ferranti. The authors give special recognition to Andil Gosine, whose critical eye, knowledge of the Caribbean and endless patience were critical in bringing this report to publication.

We thank the many men and women from the Caribbean who made this report a truly regional undertaking, including members of the National Youth Council of St. Lucia, and of Addiction Alert in Jamaica. And most important, we thank the young people from the Caribbean who shared their stories, successes, and frustrations with us with the hope that we would disseminate their word to our audience. We hope that we have met your expectations.

ACRONYMS

AIDS	acquired immune deficiency syndrome
AZT	azidovudine
CAREC	Caribbean Epidemiology Center
CARICOM	Caribbean Community
CEE	Common Entrance Exam
CGCED	Caribbean Group for Cooperation and Economic Development
CIDA	Canadian International Development Agency
COSHSOD	Commission for Human and Social Development
CPI	Consumer Protection Index
CXC	Caribbean Examinations Council
CYP	Commonwealth Youth Programme
DFID	Department for International Development (United Kingdom)
ECLAC	Economic Commission for Latin America and the Caribbean
GDP	gross domestic product
HEART	Human Employment and Resource Training
HIV	human immunodeficiency virus
ILO	International Labour Organisation
IMF	International Monetary Fund
LAC	Latin America and the Caribbean
LSMS	Living Standards Measurement Study
MLG	Ministry of Local Government (Jamaica)
NGO	nongovernmental organization
NTA	National Training Agency
NYC	National Youth Council
OECS	Organization of Eastern Caribbean States
PAHO	Pan American Health Organization
PIOJ	Planning Institute of Jamaica
SERVOL	Service Volunteered for All
STI	sexually transmitted infection
U.N.	United Nations
UNAIDS	Joint United Nations Programme on HIV/AIDS
UNDCP	United Nations International Drug Control Programme
UNDP	United Nations Development Programme
UNESCO	United Nations Educational, Scientific, and Cultural Organization
UNFPA	United Nations Population Fund
UNICEF	United Nations Children's Fund
USAID	United States Agency for International Development

EXECUTIVE SUMMARY

Introduction

This report responds to the growing concern over issues facing Caribbean youth today and, specifically, to a request made by the Caribbean Group for Cooperation and Economic Development (CGCED) to report on the subject of youth at the Sixteenth CGCED Conference held in June 2002. Much has been written about the problems plaguing Caribbean youth, but much less is known about the underlying causes of those problems and what should be done about them. This report attempts to contribute to the debate and discussion on these questions.

Caribbean youth are generally happy and healthy. They attend school, participate in social and cultural events, enjoy the loving support of a family and peers, and plan for the future. Youth played a critical role in the birth of the politically independent Caribbean, and very many of them continue to overcome remarkable odds to achieve lofty personal and professional goals. However, factors are present in the Caribbean that have the potential to disrupt the process of positive youth development. This report focuses on those who are at risk of deviating or who have already deviated from healthy behaviors.

The objectives of this report are threefold. It aims to (1) identify the risk and protective factors and determinants of youth behaviors and development, (2) demonstrate that the negative behaviors of youth are costly not only to the youth themselves but to society as a whole, and (3) identify key intervention points for youth development, taking into account identified risk and protective factors for the Caribbean. The report is based mainly on the following data sources: a Pan American Health Organization (PAHO) dataset (1997–99) on the behaviors of school-going adolescents from nine Caribbean Community (CARICOM) countries; focus groups and in-depth interviews carried out in the Dominican Republic and Saint Lucia in 2002; household or labor force surveys (1995–99) for Saint Lucia, Guyana, the Dominican Republic, and Jamaica; and consultations on study findings with stakeholders from the Dominican Republic and the English-speaking Caribbean.

This report relies on data sources and studies from as many Caribbean countries as possible, but it focuses on the Bank's client countries, these being the Organization of Eastern Caribbean

States (OECS), Belize, the Dominican Republic, Guyana, Haiti, Jamaica, Suriname, and Trinidad and Tobago. It places less focus on Haiti because of socioeconomic disparities between Haiti and its neighboring Caribbean countries.

Conceptual Framework

For the purposes of this study, *youth* is defined as spanning the adolescent period from 10 to 24 years of age. *Youth or adolescent development* thus refers to the physical, social, and emotional processes of maturation that occur during the 10- to 24-year age period. The adolescent period represents the transition from childhood to adulthood, with biological processes riving the initiation of adolescence and societal factors largely determining the initiation of adulthood.

This study uses an "ecological" framework to demonstrate the linkages between (a) the underlying risk and protective factors of youth behaviors, (b) youth outcomes, and (c) subsequent adult outcomes. It is termed "ecological" because the framework shows the relationship between the individual adolescent and his or her environment. *Risk factors* are those factors that increase the likelihood of experiencing negative outcomes. *Protective factors* counterbalance the risk factors.

Risk and protective factors exist at three levels: at the level of the *individual*, the *microenvironment* (comprising family, social networks, peers and role models, community, and neighborhood), and the *macroenvironment* (including mass media, the economy, public institutions, cultural and historical background, and social norms on gender). A simplistic version of the framework shows that risk and protective factors affect youth outcomes, which in turn shape the kind of adults the youth will become. Negative risk outcomes can, in turn, become risk factors.

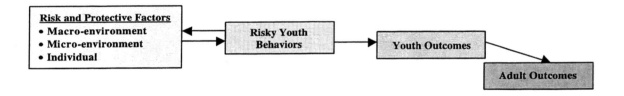

Key Findings

Although the Caribbean Is Culturally Diverse, Many Negative Youth Outcomes Are Common Across Countries and Particular to the Caribbean Region.

Despite historical, political, cultural, and linguistic diversity, the negative outcomes observed among Caribbean youth are quite similar. These include early sexual initiation, HIV/AIDS, sexual and physical abuse, school leaving (dropout and exit), unemployment, crime and violence, substance abuse and drug dealing, and social exclusion. Negative outcomes that are particular to Caribbean countries are briefly described below.

- *Sexual and physical abuse is high in the Caribbean and socially accepted in many Caribbean countries.* Corporal punishment continues to be widespread in Caribbean schools and homes, particularly among boys. And according to the nine-country CARICOM study, 1 in 10 school-going adolescents have been sexually abused. The high incidence of sexual abuse among Caribbean boys stands out in comparison to other countries. Even more noteworthy is the "disturbing pattern of cultural 'normalcy' in child and physical and sexual abuse" in the Caribbean (Barrow 2001).
- *The onset of sexual initiation in the Caribbean is the earliest in the world* (with the exception of Africa, where early sexual experiences take place within marriage). Early sexual debut is known to predispose young people to early pregnancy, HIV/AIDS, and other sexually transmitted infections (STIs).

- *The region has the highest incidence of HIV/AIDS outside of Africa*—and youth are an at-risk group. Among other things, HIV/AIDS is linked to cultural values about sexuality that are particular to the Caribbean.
- *The incidence of rage among young people is extremely high:* 40 percent of school-going CARICOM students reported feelings of rage. High rates of sexual abuse and physical abuse among children likely play out in rage among young people, which can affect their school performance and lead to violence.
- *Youth unemployment is especially elevated in some Caribbean countries.* According to World Development Indicators from 1996 to 1998, St. Lucia had the highest youth unemployment rate in the Americas, followed by Jamaica. In the Caribbean, St. Lucia, followed by Dominica, St. Vincent and the Grenadines, and Jamaica, have the highest youth unemployment rates.
- In contrast to the United States, which has high levels of youth violence, *the proportion of Caribbean adolescent males who carry firearms is extremely high.* Fully one-fifth of students had carried a weapon to school in the 30 days previous to the survey, and nearly as many had been in a fight using weapons. *Gang violence is also high in the Caribbean,* with 20 percent of male students and 12 percent of female students at one point having belonged to a gang.
- Although data on drug use are scanty, anecdotal evidence suggests a *widespread social acceptance of alcohol and marijuana in some Caribbean countries,* among both in-school and out-of-school youth. Out-of-school youth aged 13 to 19 years are most at risk of substance abuse as well as drug dealing (Barker 1995). Further complicating the situation, the Caribbean is a major trans-shipment point for drugs entering the United States and Europe.

Costs of Risky Adolescent Behavior Are High.

Problems plaguing Caribbean youth are costly. Although it is impossible to put a value on a human life or on the range of positive and negative externalities generated by youth, rough estimates show that losses to society from risky youth behaviors such as teen pregnancy, school leaving, crime, and HIV/AIDS—both in terms of direct expenditures and forgone productivity—reach into the billions of dollars. Some rough calculations are as follows:

- A single cohort of adolescent mothers is estimated to cost society, in terms of forgone benefits from alternative uses of resources, more than US$2 million in St. Kitts and Nevis.
- School leavers in Guyana forgo hundreds of thousands of dollars in net earnings over their lifetimes, costing the state thousands of dollars in lost income.
- Youth crime and violence in St. Lucia generates more than US$3 million in lost benefits to society and US$7.7 million in lost benefits to private individuals *annually.*
- A 1 percent decrease in youth crime would increase tourist receipts by 4 percent in Jamaica and by 2.3 percent in the Bahamas.
- The financial loss to society due to AIDS deaths among those who contracted AIDS during adolescence ranges from 0.01 percent of gross domestic product (GDP) in Suriname and Antigua and Barbuda to 0.17 percent of GDP in the Bahamas in just the year 2000.
- If female youth unemployment were reduced to the level of adult unemployment, GDP would be higher by a range of 0.4 percent in Antigua and Barbuda and 2.9 percent in Jamaica.

Youth Are Not the Problem.

Youth are not the problem but a product of their micro- and macroenvironments. For the most part, they rationally react to the situation in which they find themselves. Drug dealing, for example, would be rational for a young person if no other forms of employment existed, the family needed money, and the drug lord provided protection and a sense of belonging. Evidence from this study suggests that in the Caribbean, the following factors are the most important in determining the outcomes of youth:

- *Family:* The family is both the strongest protective factor and the strongest risk factor for youth behavior and outcomes. It is protective in that family connectedness, appropriate levels of parental discipline, moral guidance, protection from dangers in the adult world, and economic support allow young people to acquire personal and social skills while young. Conversely, parental displays of negative behaviors (substance abuse, violence); physical, sexual, and emotional abuse by family members; and the absence of parental guidance and support are risk factors.
- *Schools:* Connectedness to schools is highly protective against all risky behaviors, including using drugs and alcohol and engaging in violent or sexual activity. For example, among school-going adolescents, the probability of sexual behavior falls by 30 percentage points for boys and 60 percentage points for girls if they are connected to schools. Conversely, the school system can have devastating effects on those youth with low academic achievement by not granting them a place in school and, as a corollary, making them feel socially excluded and "worthless."
- *Poverty:* Young people in disadvantaged situations are often forced to find work and have few options except informal sector work, drug trade, or prostitution. Parents— particularly single parents—are more likely to be absent from the household and frequently leave youth and children unattended and unsupervised. Young girls in some countries—sometimes at the encouragement of their mothers—will engage in opportunistic sex to relieve poverty and contribute to household income. And childbearing is still used a strategy for gaining economic support in countries like Jamaica. Last, income inequality—which is demonstrated by the presence of drug dons, foreign tourists, and the media—encourages the engagement of youth in "easy money" activities, including drugs and commercial sex work.
- *Gender:* Gender is a central risk factor in Caribbean societies. Almost all children in Jamaica and St. Lucia, for example, are born out of wedlock, which means that many fathers are absent from the lives of their children. The exclusionary nature of fathering dates back to slavery, when men were not permitted to play the role of spouse and father. At the same time, social norms promote sexual prowess and multifathering among men. These norms have important intergenerational effects. Children of absent fathers are more likely to fare poorly in school. And men's inability to provide economic support means that women often raise children on their own, leading to greater levels of poverty and vulnerability among these women and their children.

A key message that arises out of research findings is the *interconnectedness of factors that predispose risky behavior and outcomes.* Empirical analysis of risk and protective factors carried out using the nine-country CARICOM data demonstrates the complex interrelations among family, school, and community factors in the microenvironment. Study results also show that changing any one of the risk factors will improve outcomes. These findings are consistent with the international evidence.

Many Youth Programs Exist, but Little Is Known about Their Effectiveness.
Much is being done in the area of youth development, with government and the nongovernmental organization (NGO) sector both active in different ways. Innovative private sector and private-public sector initiatives for youth also look promising. At the regional level, CARICOM's Regional Strategy for Youth Development represents an important step in placing youth on the regional agenda. The CYP has also made significant progress in assisting Caribbean countries to develop youth policies and building a cadre of youth and professional staff qualified to work on youth

issues. As for international donor support, the United Nations Children's Fund (UNICEF) is playing a leading role in youth development. In particular, its strategy to promote cross-institutional collaboration through community multipurpose youth hubs appears to be promising. But limited information on the situation of youth themselves—particularly out-of-school youth who are unattached to formal institutions—and on the nature and effectiveness of the multitude of programs that exist makes evaluation and informed planning difficult. The cross-cutting nature of youth, which implies a need for effective coordination across institutional lines, presents an additional challenge.

Moving Forward: Youth Development Principles and Actions

Although the transitional period from childhood to adulthood is unquestionably a challenge for many, the majority of Caribbean youth make the transition unencumbered. Yet the report demonstrates that there are serious social and economic consequences associated with not addressing the minority group of youth who are at risk of negative behaviors or are suffering the impact of their negative circumstances—not only for the youth themselves and their families, but for society at large. This situation thus calls for decisive action of the part of Caribbean policymakers and governments in the area of youth development.

Building on available research and practice, the report puts forward a set of principles to guide youth development efforts in Caribbean states in both the macro- and microenvironments. These include (a) taking a life-cycle, age-specific approach; (b) ensuring selectivity and focus; (c) taking an asset-based approach; (d) establishing comprehensive long-term supports for youth; and (e) taking intersectoral integrated approaches to youth development.

As for specific policy recommendations, programs and policies as well as specific actions must be context specific, that is, based on the nature and acuteness of the youth issues faced by each country as well as the institutional context. But some specific recommendations pertaining to the Caribbean include:

- *Reforming the education system and maximizing the protective effects of schools* by improving access and retention, improving the quality of education, eliminating corporal punishment, using educational activities and campaigns to reduce violence and promote conflict resolution, and institutionalizing permanent, school-based information and education campaigns on sexual abuse and exploitation.
- *Upgrading the public health care system* by establishing new protocols, tools, and techniques for reaching youth and their families, including: developing mental health approaches, upgrading the skills of existing health professionals, training graduates on new protocols, and ensuring that protocols include confidentiality and gender-differentiated services. It is important to ensure that the nursing and medical professions play a role in condemning sexual and physical abuse of children and adolescents and putting the issue on the public health agenda.
- *Institutionalizing national-level mentoring systems for at-risk youth* by identifying existing effective programs and creating incentives for NGOs and the private sector to expand these programs to the national level.
- *Reforming and strengthening legal, judicial, and policing systems* by improving juvenile justice (review and harmonization of laws, strengthening of family courts, training of legal practitioners, modernizing of the courts, and use of alternative custodial sentences), increasing the control of weapons, and reforming the police.
- *Using the media and social marketing* to change norms and values related to the following key risk areas for youth: sexual abuse and exploitation, early sexual initiation, corporal punishment and physical abuse, and alcohol consumption and drug use. Use social marketing techniques(which draw on commercial marketing principles) to increase the effectiveness of communication and education techniques.

- *Making families and fathers a top public policy issue:* Put in place incentives to make parents accountable for their children (legal measures, tax breaks) and use the education system, the public health system, and the media to teach at-risk parents fundamental parenting skills; put in place incentives to increase fathers' rights to and responsibilities for their children.
- *Strengthening community and neighborhood supports to adolescents and their families* by establishing competitive "youth funds" to finance innovative NGO and community-based initiatives for youth (e.g., as part of social development funds).

INTRODUCTION

I

Background and Justification

There is a growing concern among the public and policymakers alike over the situation of Caribbean youth today. Most youth are doing well; the majority of young people in the Caribbean do not engage in violent activities, participate in illicit drug trade, or drop out of school. But there is increasing recognition of those who are not able to overcome the challenges presented to them by their environment. Terms such as "in crisis," "plight," and "in peril" are commonly used in reference to Caribbean youth (1997, Williams 2002). The concerns that have been raised over and over again in the discourses and literature on youth in the Caribbean include the spread of AIDS among young people, the threat to well-being by early initiation into sexual activity and teenage pregnancy, the pervasive youth unemployment, the inequality of education, the involvement of youth in drug trade and crime and violence as an alternative to unemployment and poverty, and the social exclusion of youth. The CYP's publication "Tomorrow's Adults: A Situational Analysis of Youth in the Commonwealth Caribbean" notes that although youth would legally be adults from the age of 18 in most countries, many young people in the Caribbean are denied passage into adulthood as a result of labor market constraints, lack of participation in decisionmaking processes, constraints to ownership of property and goods, and lack of status and role in society (Danns, Henry, and LaFleur 1997).

Caribbean youth issues have emerged during volatile macroeconomic conditions. Over the last two decades, many Caribbean nations experienced economic decline and stagnation resulting from a loss of their preferential treatment in agriculture markets, depressed market for minerals, losses due to lack of market diversification, stagnation of the manufacturing sector in the face of increased competition, and increasing vulnerability of the tourism sector. Several countries thus have implemented structural adjustment and stabilization programs, with corollary cutbacks in health, education, housing, and social welfare programs. More recently, global economic recession, debt service obligations, and declines in development assistance have prevented many Caribbean nations from economic recovery and growth.

Is it true that many youth in the Caribbean are at risk? Is the situation of Caribbean youth significantly different from that in other countries in the face of economic downturn and stagnation? Although a broad term, *at risk* generally refers to youth who face "environmental, social and family conditions that [potentially] hinder their personal development and their successful integration into society as productive citizens" (Barker and Fontes 1996). For most youth worldwide, the critical transition period from childhood to young adulthood is delicate and challenging, and it hinges on the adequate support and guidance from family, schools, and society at large (Feldman and Elliott 1997). The literature on youth in the Caribbean and the findings of this report suggest that negative youth outcomes are a result of failures on the part of families, government, and society as a whole to provide the appropriate and adequate supports for young people to grow into responsible and productive adults.

There has been much debate and discussion on the challenges Caribbean youth face, but relatively little has been done to gain an understanding of the nature of their problems, the underlying causes of youth risks and behaviors, and the corollary policies and programs required to address the issues. Youth development and youth at risk have been on the agendas of most Caribbean governments for some time. According to Huggins (1998), most Caribbean countries have identified youth as a target for social development and welfare planning, having set up youth desks and departments in government, assigned public resources for youth, and funded programs specifically for youth (cited in Alexis 2000). However, although attention has been dedicated to youth, limited empirical analysis and evaluation have been carried out to underpin these programs (Alexis 2000). The focus of youth programs has been on leisure and service to the community rather than developing a good understanding of the needs of and challenges faced by youth and how meeting these needs and addressing these challenges can lead to the overall economic and social development of societies as a whole in the Caribbean.

Recognizing the importance of youth issues and the need for an improved empirical basis for youth programs, governments in the Caribbean have requested the Bank's assistance to better understand the nature of youth issues and what needs to be done to improve the conditions for youth; examine the costs of *not* investing in youth, given competing demands for resources; and identify the role of the state and other actors in providing services to youth. Specifically, in 2000, the Caribbean Group for Cooperation and Economic Development (CGCED) selected "youth" as one of the featured topics at its June 2002 meeting. This report serves as the World Bank's main contribution to youth development for the June meeting.

Objectives, Approach, and Data Sources
Objectives
This document has three specific research objectives: (1) to identify the risk and protective factors that affect youth development in the Caribbean, (2) to demonstrate that the issues facing Caribbean youth are costly not only to themselves but to society as a whole, and (3) to identify key intervention points for youth development, taking into account identified risk and protective factors

Data and Methodology
A youth development framework, based on the public health literature and adapted to the Caribbean, serves as the organizing structure to the report. This framework organizes the influences of youth development by identifying risk and protective factors within the macroenvironment, the microenvironment (peers, family, and community), and the individual him- or herself.

For the analysis, the report draws on both original data collection and analysis and a review of existing literature. The primary data sources were

▪ Pan American Health Organization (PAHO) health data (1997–99): A cross-sectional dataset from nine Caribbean Community (CARICOM) countries (Antigua and Barbuda, the Bahamas, Barbados, British Virgin Islands, Dominica, Grenada, Guyana, Jamaica, and

St. Lucia[1]) that includes information on youth behaviors and their causes (hereafter referred to as the nine-country CARICOM study). Statisticians at the ministries of health in each country collected the school-based data. Sample size was representative of school-going teenagers within each country, which does not represent all youth because many leave school before graduation.

▨ *Focus groups and in-depth interviews from the Dominican Republic and St. Lucia (2002):* Qualitative data were collected from 26 focus group discussions with young men and women and 27 in-depth, semistructured interviews with youth experts in the Dominican Republic and St. Lucia. Sixteen focus groups were made up of 6 to 10 youth aged 14 to 24 years who were considered at risk of engaging in unhealthy behaviors or who currently do engage in such behaviors. The samples were drawn from juvenile detention centers, church groups, community groups, schools, and a wide range of youth in both rural and urban areas of the countries. The remaining focus groups were youth not at risk (control groups) and adult parents or peers of youth. Discussions with all the focus groups emphasized preconditions that lead to unhealthy youth behavior and the motivation for participation in such behavior. In St. Lucia, focus groups were also held with the parents and adult peers of the at-risk youth. The structured interviews with youth experts served for triangulation and to better understand the breach between the understanding of those who work with youth and the youth themselves.

▨ *Household or labor force surveys (1995–99):* Household or labor force surveys for St. Lucia (1995), Guyana (1999), the Dominican Republic (1998), and Jamaica (1998) were used to cost-out the youth behaviors. Country selection was based solely on the availability of data.

Datasets are used for different purposes throughout the report. The analysis of risk and protective factors was based on the qualitative data and econometric analysis of the PAHO data. The analysis of the cost of risky youth behavior relied on household and labor force surveys as well as databases of international organizations including PAHO, the International Labour Organisation (ILO), and the United Nations (U.N.). The review of programs and the existing network for youth support in the Caribbean relied on the semistructured interviews. All sections were heavily supported with existing literature.

Caribbean Context
Territorial Scope

Definitions of the territorial scope of the Caribbean vary. According to the World Bank (2000a), the "wider" Caribbean region includes

▨ the sovereign-state members of CARICOM, including both island-nations (Antigua and Barbuda, the Bahamas, Barbados, Dominica, Grenada, Haiti, Jamaica, Montserrat, St. Kitts and Nevis, St. Lucia, St. Vincent and the Grenadines, and Trinidad and Tobago) and the mainland countries of Belize in Central America and Guyana and Suriname in South America;

▨ Spanish-speaking Cuba and the Dominican Republic;

▨ the semiautonomous states of the Kingdom of the Netherlands (Aruba and the Netherlands Antilles islands of Bonaire, Curaçao, St. Martin, St. Eustatius, and Saba);

▨ the British Overseas Territories, that is, Anguilla, Bermuda, the British Virgin Islands, the Cayman Islands, and the Turks and Caicos Islands;

▨ the U.S. commonwealth of Puerto Rico and territory of the U.S. Virgin Islands; and

▨ The territories of the French Republic consisting of French Guyana, St. Martin, Saint-Pierre and Miquelon, Guadeloupe, and Martinique.

---

1. The survey was a collaborative effort between the ministries of health in the nine countries, PAHO, and the World Health Organization (WHO) Collaborating Center in Adolescent Health at the University of Minnesota, Minneapolis.

The Caribbean is a multiethnic region with many cultural differences. There are English-speaking countries (e.g., Trinidad and Tobago), Spanish-speaking countries (e.g., the Dominican Republic), French-speaking countries (e.g., Haiti), and Dutch-speaking countries (e.g., Suriname). The majority of the population is of African descent, although there are also people of European, Hispanic, and East and South Asian ancestry (e.g., Indians in Trinidad and Tobago and Guyana).

The mainland states of Belize, Guyana, and Suriname, which by virtue of language and heritage form part of the Caribbean region, are much larger in land mass than the island states of the Caribbean: Belize (29,963 square kilometers; population, 215,000), Guyana (219,470 square kilometers; population, 813,000), and Suriname (163,820 square kilometers; population, 437,000). The island states of the Caribbean vary in size and population from Anguilla (91 square kilometers; population, 8,000) to Jamaica (11,424 square kilometers; population, 2,447,000).

Historically, the Caribbean region has been strongly influenced by Europe and the United States. Many of the English-speaking Caribbean countries have modeled their educational, legal, and political systems on those of the United Kingdom. The countries of the English-speaking Caribbean have a combined population of around 6.7 million scattered over the Caribbean Sea, whose farthest points span about 3,500 kilometers between the coast of Belize and Guyana. The Bahamas and the Dominican Republic are economically reliant on the United States. France and the Netherlands also have strong links with some of the non-English speaking countries, for example Martinique and Curaçao. Therefore, there has been much migration from these countries to the Caribbean. The Caribbean is a major tourist destination, attracting visitors from many parts of the world. Similarly, over the past 40 years, for economic reasons, many Caribbean citizens have migrated, primarily to the United States, Canada, and the United Kingdom. There is also much business travel within and outside the Caribbean.

For the purposes of this report, the Caribbean area of focus includes the Bank's client countries: these being the Organization of Eastern Caribbean States (OECS) (Anguilla, Antigua and Barbuda, the British Virgin Islands, Dominica, Grenada, Montserrat, St. Kitts and Nevis, St. Lucia, St. Vincent and the Grenadines), as well as Belize, the Dominican Republic, Guyana, Haiti, Jamaica, Suriname, and Trinidad and Tobago. However, given the disparity in socioeconomic conditions between Haiti and its Caribbean neighbors, limited focus is placed on that country.

Demographics of Caribbean Youth

Caribbean youth make up about 30 percent of the population (see table 1.1), with data for available countries indicating that St. Lucia has the highest proportion of youth aged 10 to 24 years (34 percent) and St. Kitts and Nevis having the lowest proportion (24 percent).

REPORT ORGANIZATION

The report is organized as follows: Subsequent to this introductory chapter, Chapter two provides a framework for analyzing youth development, presenting an integrative model of risk and protective factors for youth development and subsequent adult health and well-being in the context of the Caribbean. Chapter three reviews negative outcomes observed among Caribbean youth. Chapter four presents findings of the analysis of risk and protective factors of negative youth outcomes based on qualitative and quantitative analysis of Caribbean data and information, as well as other sources. Chapter five puts forward an argument for investing in youth by presenting an analysis of cost estimations of the risky behaviors associated with youth. Chapter six presents a discussion on policies and programming related to youth in the Caribbean. And finally, chapter seven provides conclusions, a proposed strategy, and key policy entry points.

TABLE 1-1: TOTAL POPULATION BY AGE GROUP FOR SELECTED CARIBBEAN COUNTRIES

Age group	St. Vincent and the Grenadines Year 2000 % of total population	St. Vincent and the Grenadines Year 2000 Population by age group	St. Kitts and Nevis Year 2000 % of total population	St. Kitts and Nevis Year 2000 Population by age group	Grenada Year 2000 % of total population	Grenada Year 2000 Population by age group	Dominican Republic Year 1998 % of total population	Dominican Republic Year 1998 Population by age group	Jamaica Year 1997 % of total population	Jamaica Year 1997 Population by age group	Guyana Year 1999 % of total population	Guyana Year 1999 Population by age group	St. Lucia Year 1995 % of total population	St. Lucia Year 1995 Population by age group	Barbados Year 1995 % of total population	Barbados Year 1995 Population by age group
0–4	11.7	13,455	7.8	3,198	10.0	9,800	11.7	968,218	11.5	293,199	12.1	103,909	9.1	13,235	7.5	19,899
5–9	13.9	15,985	9.9	4,049	11.9	11,662	13.0	1,073,871	11.7	298,052	12.3	105,193	12.4	18,035	8.2	21,742
10–14	12.4	14,260	9.3	3,823	13.4	13,132	11.6	953,360	11.5	293,965	11.2	96,120	12.7	18,471	8.3	22,022
15–19	11.2	12,880	8.2	3,352	11.2	10,976	10.6	876,596	9.6	243,907	10.0	85,849	12.2	17,744	9.1	24,205
20–24	8.8	10,120	6.6	2,686	7.6	7,448	8.9	735,449	8.4	214,281	8.6	73,609	9.1	13,235	8.6	22,726
25–29	6.9	7,935	7.4	3,045	6.5	6,370	7.8	644,653	8.6	219,389	8.6	73,951	8.4	12,217	9.3	24,539
30–34	7.4	8,510	7.6	3116	6.4	6,272	7.4	609,985	7.3	185,420	7.2	61,198	6.2	9,017	8.8	23,350
35–39	5.9	6,785	8.9	3,659	7.4	7,252	5.9	488,649	6.2	157,837	7.4	63,252	7.1	10,326	7.4	19,524
40–44	5.0	5,750	5.8	2,358	5.1	4,998	5.0	409,408	4.5	115,952	6.3	53,666	3.9	5,672	5.9	15,553
45–49	1.7	1,955	6.4	2,624	3.5	3,430	4.1	340,073	3.8	980,74	4.6	38,944	3.7	5,381	4.2	11,078
50–54	3.4	3,910	3.3	1,343	2.9	2,842	3.5	290,548	3.1	79,429	3.3	28,588	3.3	4,800	3.8	10,152
55–59	2.5	2,875	2.8	1,138	2.8	2,744	2.6	215,435	3.1	79,940	2.3	19,601	2.2	3,200	3.4	8,927
60–64	3.5	4,025	3.8	1,538	3.3	3,234	2.6	213,784	3.0	76,620	2.0	17,461	2.5	3,636	3.9	9,157
65+	5.7	6,555	12.4	5,084	8.0	7,840	5.3	434,171	7.8	197,935	4.0	34,579	7.2	10,472	11.8	31,264
Total	100.0	115000	100.0	41,010	100.0	98,000	100.0	8,254,200	100.0	2,554,000	100.0	855,920	100.0	145,440	100	264,137

Sources: World Development Indicators (World Bank 1997), PAHO Core Health Data System 2000, Living Standards Measurement Study (LSMS) (World Bank 1997–99)

2

FRAMEWORK FOR ANALYZING CARIBBEAN YOUTH

Definitions

Youth

The literature is replete with caution on the use of a chronological age to distinguish phases of the life cycle. The definition of youth depends on the sectoral and cultural context; for example, health specialists may refer to youth as the pubescent period, which begins at different ages in different countries, and labor ministries may use the minimum work age as the age when youth begins. The U.N. definition of youth is 15 to 24 years old. The majority of youth policies in the Caribbean, however, see youth as beginning at age 15 and ending at 30 years (Alexis 2000). The reason for this extended period of youth in the Caribbean is the extremely high rate of youth unemployment that prevents young people from attaining adult status (Danns, Henry, and LaFleur 1997).

For the purposes of this study, youth is defined as spanning the adolescent period between 10 and 24 years of age, with "youth" and "adolescents" being used interchangeably.[2] Adolescence encompasses the transition from childhood to adulthood. Biological processes drive the initiation of adolescence, its onset being defined by puberty (Feldmen and Elliott 1997). In contrast, societal factors largely determine the initiation of adulthood. Because of the broad period it encompasses, adolescence can be divided into three subcategories: early adolescence (ages 10 to 14), during which intense physical and social changes corresponding with puberty take place; middle adolescence (ages 15 to 17), during which young people become increasingly independent; and late adolescence (ages 17 to mid-20s), which applies to those who for social or other reasons delay entry into adulthood (Feldmen and Elliott 1997).

---

2. The definition of youth used in this report deviates from that of the U.N. and the Caribbean by lowering the onset of youth to age 10. This is necessary because of the ecological approach of the model, which identifies influences of youth behavior that begin as early as age 10.

Youth Development

Youth or adolescent development refers to the physical, social, and emotional processes of maturation that occur during the 10- to 24-year age period. The elements of this developmental period
include pubertal maturation, cognitive development, ability to understand a future time perspective,
ability to extrapolate, experimentation (including gender role experimentation), and moral development (see box 2-1).

Engaging in prosocial behaviors and avoiding health-compromising and future jeopardizing
behaviors lead to positive youth development (Roth et al. 1998). A sense of industry and competency, a feeling of connectedness to others and society, a belief in controlling one's fate, and a
stable identity are elements of positive development in adolescence. Risk-taking behaviors predispose youth to negative outcomes (e.g., unprotected intercourse is a health risk behavior that predisposes to sexually transmitted infections [STIs] and unwanted pregnancy). The outcomes of
these risk behaviors (e.g., early, nonmarital childbearing; early school leaving; drug addiction;
violence; etc.) compromise a young person's future and can have high societal costs in the short
and long term.

Factors Contributing to Youth Development

While research and policy on youth have tended to focus on the behavioral aspects of youth development, recent work has shifted to the underlying causes of these behaviors (World Bank 2000b).
Risk factors, also referred to as risk antecedents, are those factors that increase the likelihood of
experiencing negative outcomes (Resnick and Hojat 1997). Factors predisposing negative outcomes may be individual (e.g., aggressive temperament), familial (e.g., substance-abusing families,
familial mental illness), or environmental (e.g., high crime and violence neighborhoods).

BOX 2-1: ELEMENTS OF ADOLESCENT DEVELOPMENT

- **Pubertal Maturation,** which include three key changes: (a) the development of adult reproductive capabili-
  ties; (b) the establishment of sexual dimorphism; and (c) the completion of organ system maturation.
- **Cognitive development,** including a shift in cognition from *concrete thinking* to the *formal operations* of adolescence, which allow for abstract reasoning skills as well as a capacity for future time perspective, and thus
  the capability of understanding the long-as well as short-term consequences of one's behavior.
- **Extrapolation and Experimentation,** which represents a shift from concrete to abstract operational
  thought, and the increased ability to apply the lessons of daily life. *Extrapolation* is the capacity to take the
  lessons learned from past experiences and apply them to new situations. The mechanism by which this
  aspect of cognition develops is through *experimentation.* Whether it is through cigarette smoking, provocative
  clothing, a new hairstyle, or sexual behavior, experimentation is a concrete, experiential way of learning
  compared, for example, to information learned at school which is more abstract when one studies the experiences of others. It is through a similar process of role experimentations that one learns and internalizes
  gender appropriate behavior.
- **Moral development:** Moral development represents a process through which individuals mature in dealing
  with complex value-based decisions. Kohlberg (1981) defined six stages through which individuals progress as
  they move from early childhood to adulthood: (a) the first stage being "punishment/obedience", in which a
  child is motivated to behave in a certain way because he believes that if he does not do so he will be punished; (b) a second in which a child's actions are is motivated by self-gain; (c) a third stage, in which behavior
  is based on a desire to be liked; (d) a fourth stage in which maintenance of social order, fixed rules, and
  authority are the major motivations for behavior; (e) a fifth stage in which moral reasoning is based on a
  notion of social contract: "the greatest good for the greatest number."; and (f) the last and highest level in
  which decisions are based on a "universal ethical principle" or justice.

Counterbalancing such risks are the protective factors (Blum 1998) that likewise arise from the individual, familial, and social environments in which a young person lives.[3] For example, individual characteristics that have been repeatedly found to be protective include social skills, intelligence, and a belief in a higher power beyond oneself. Protective family characteristics include a caring parent, an authoritative parenting style, and smaller family size. Likewise, social environments associated with reduced risk include caring nonfamilial adults, collective self-efficacy, and neighborhood engagement. Thus, as a dynamic process, one must concurrently consider both the factors that predispose to vulnerability and those that protect (direct effect) or buffer (indirect or mediated effect) a young person from harm.

It is important to note, however, that although risk and protective factors aid in understanding underlying causes of behaviors, the subjective experiences of adolescents and youth are tremendously varied. Although the odds of negative behaviors are much higher for those individuals who have many risk factors, not all succumb. The concept of resilience may help to explain the reasons why youth outcomes are not foreordained. Resilience refers to the self-righting capacity of an individual to bounce back and keep going. It implies resistance to threat but not invincibility (Garmezy 1991) or invulnerability (Garmezy 1985). Rutter (1993) suggests that resilience is interactive with vulnerabilities. That is, resilience is developmental in nature, stemming from biology and experiences earlier in life, and protective factors may operate in different ways at different stages of development.

Conceptual Framework

Figure 2-1 provides the conceptual framework used in this report to discuss underlying protective and risk factors associated with youth outcomes and behaviors and their subsequent adult outcomes. It is based on an "ecological" model of human development that sees human development and youth development taking place in overlapping interrelated spheres that include home, family, school, and community (Blum 2002). The framework, which was constructed for the Caribbean based on what is known about the risks Caribbean adolescents face and their probable underlying causes, outlines risk and protective categories at three levels: the macroenvironment, the microenvironment, and the individual. Macro-level factors are the macro systems and institutions that affect an individual but with which the individual does not have direct contact, whereas the microenvironment refers to institutions and individuals with which the adolescent interacts on a personal basis—it refers to his or her space or sphere of interaction. The inherent and learned characteristics that an individual possesses also act as protective or risk factors independently or by interaction with micro- and macroenvironmental factors. Risk and protective factors are those forces that underlie or determine adolescent behavior. Adolescent behavior, risk-taking or otherwise, determines adult outcomes later in life. All of these concepts are briefly discussed in turn.

Macroenvironmental Factors

The macroenvironment represents the "distal contexts of adolescence" (Feldman and Elliott 1997), that is, the adolescent's macroenvironment or context that is detached from him or her. Risk and protective factors related to the macroenvironment include the state of the national economy, poverty and inequality levels, the institutional framework (public institutions, policy and legal frameworks), political realities, the cultural and historical background, the media, gender (values, behavioral norms, and customs), and social exclusion. For example:

- The **mass media,** including television, radio, videos, movies, music, newspapers, and magazines, play formative roles in the lives of youth worldwide (Feldman and Elliott 1997), and the Caribbean is no exception. The media serve to teach youth and influences their beliefs, values, social and political views, attitudes, and behaviors, both positive and negative.

---

3. Patterson and Blum (1996) refer to "resources," Benson (1997) refers to "assets," and Masten and Reed (2000) refer to "resilience" as countering the risk factors.

FIGURE 2-1: CARRIBBEAN FRAMEWORK OF RISK AND PROTECTIVE FACTORS FOR ADOLESCENT AND SUBSEQUENT ADULT DEVELOPMENT

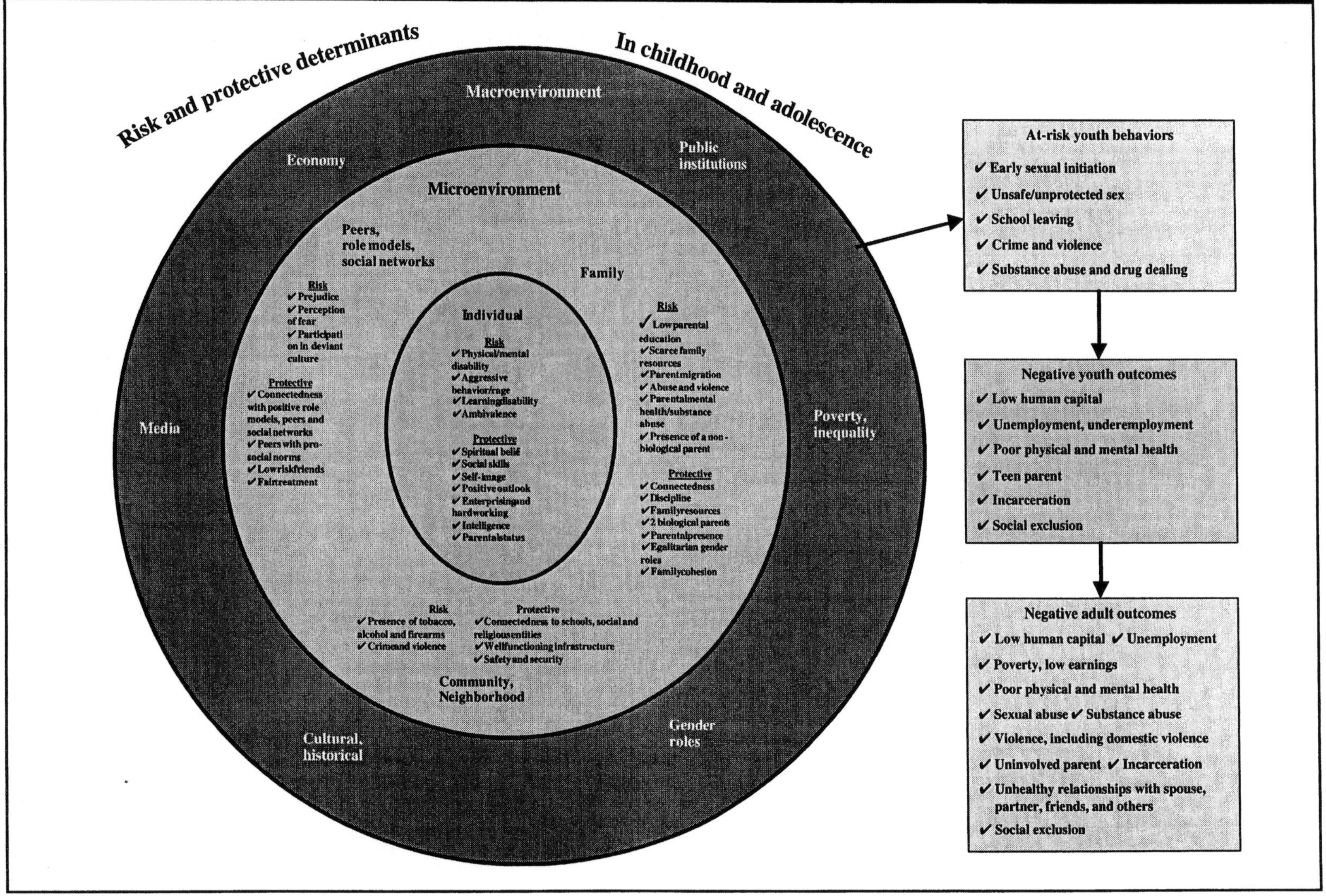

At-risk youth behaviors
- ✓ Early sexual initiation
- ✓ Unsafe/unprotected sex
- ✓ School leaving
- ✓ Crime and violence
- ✓ Substance abuse and drug dealing

Negative youth outcomes
- ✓ Low human capital
- ✓ Unemployment, underemployment
- ✓ Poor physical and mental health
- ✓ Teen parent
- ✓ Incarceration
- ✓ Social exclusion

Negative adult outcomes
- ✓ Low human capital ✓ Unemployment
- ✓ Poverty, low earnings
- ✓ Poor physical and mental health
- ✓ Sexual abuse ✓ Substance abuse
- ✓ Violence, including domestic violence
- ✓ Uninvolved parent ✓ Incarceration
- ✓ Unhealthy relationships with spouse, partner, friends, and others
- ✓ Social exclusion

In childhood and adolescence

Risk and protective determinants

Poverty, inequality

Gender roles

Cultural, historical

Media

Economy

Public institutions

Microenvironment

Microenvironment

Peers, role models, social networks

Community, Neighborhood

Family

Individual

Individual

Risk
- ✓ Physical/mental disability
- ✓ Aggressive behavior
- ✓ Learning disability
- ✓ Ambivalence

Protective
- ✓ Spiritual belief
- ✓ Social skills
- ✓ Self-image
- ✓ Positive outlook
- ✓ Enterprising and hardworking
- ✓ Intelligence
- ✓ Parent status

Family

Risk
- ✓ Low parental education
- ✓ Scarce family resources
- ✓ Parent migration
- ✓ Abuse and violence
- ✓ Parental mental health/substance abuse
- ✓ Presence of a non-biological parent

Protective
- ✓ Connectedness
- ✓ Discipline
- ✓ Family resources
- ✓ 2 biological parents
- ✓ Parental presence
- ✓ Egalitarian gender roles
- ✓ Family cohesion

Community, Neighborhood

Risk
- ✓ Presence of tobacco, alcohol and firearms
- ✓ Crime and violence

Protective
- ✓ Connectedness to schools, social and religious entities
- ✓ Well functioning infrastructure
- ✓ Safety and security

Peers, role models, social networks

Risk
- ✓ Prejudice
- ✓ Perception of fear
- ✓ Participation in deviant culture

Protective
- ✓ Connectedness with positive role models, peers and social networks
- ✓ Peers with prosocial norms
- ✓ Low risk friends
- ✓ Fair treatment

Examples of risk-related factors related to mass media include portrayals of violence, risk-taking behavior, and sex-role stereotypes. Mass media can also be a risk factor by impeding other activities, such as schoolwork and academic performance.

▪ The state of the national economy is important in the lives of youth because it is a primary source of opportunities for youth and their families. It serves as a protective factor when it is a source of well-paid job opportunities, financial resources, and tax revenues, which provide resources for social services. However, the economy is a risk factor when it does not provide opportunities or is highly volatile and introduces high uncertainty and vulnerability into the lives of young people and their parents. This lack of opportunities, for example, is identified as a primary cause for high migration and increased involvement of young people in the drug trade. The economy is a larger challenge for youth in the Caribbean than in many other countries because of the small, island state nature of most countries in the region. Economies that are small and relatively undiversified have more difficulty smoothing exogenous economic and natural shocks and thus have a higher potential for economic contractions, job loss, and slow job creation.

▪ The nature of public institutions is another important risk/protective category operating at the macro level. Broadly, institutions are protective if they are transparent, efficient, effective, and responsive. Conversely, they present macro risk factors if they are corrupt, inefficient, and unresponsive to the needs of the populace. Education systems, health care systems, and law enforcement and judicial systems in particular are public institutions that play an important role in the lives of adolescents in that they influence access to education and academic performance, morbidity and mortality, access to reproductive and sexual health care services, and safety and security. Specific risk factors related to the health care system for adolescents, for example, include lack of access to appropriate health care services, problems regarding confidentiality of care, and lack of health care providers who specialize in serving adolescents. Protective factors related to schools include providing relevant curricula for learning academics, technical skills, and life skills; and access to peer groups, friends, mentors and organized activities for social development and emotional connection.

▪ In the area of cultural and historical background, many have argued that the British colonial legacy of many Caribbean countries has indirectly affected the youth of today by influencing family structure and maternal and paternal roles in child rearing. Weak and exclusionary public institutions are also blamed on the history of British colonialism (Trouillot 2001). The education system is a case in point: It is an example of a national institution that does not provide equal services to the majority and contributes to excluding a large segment of the youth population.[4]

▪ Gender, in the context of risk or protective factors, refers to the values, customs, and behavioral norms that account for sexual differentiation in identity and behavior. Gender is thus included as a macroenvironmental factor in that values, behavioral norms, and customs related to the differentiation of the sexes are shaped by society broadly. Gender is a risk factor, for example, if societal norms that dictate male behavior (e.g., men should be sexually promiscuous and bear many children) or female behavior (e.g., women should not enter the labor force) predispose youth (and subsequently adults) to negative outcomes. Gender is a protective factor if societal norms or culture dictate female behavior (girls should study hard) or male behavior (men should be responsible for providing for their children) predispose youth to positive outcomes.

Risk factors in the macroenvironment can act collectively to socially exclude youth as a group. Social exclusion is a multidimensional concept that has at least four characteristics: (1) exclusion from economic means, including unequal access to goods and services that determine human capital;

---

4. See chapter 4 for more details on this issue.

(2) unequal access to labor markets and social protection programs from both formal and informal institutions; (3) exclusion from participatory mechanisms that affect public service programs; and (4) unequal access to political rights and civil liberties (Gacitúa, Soto, and Davis 2001).

Microenvironmental Factors

The micro-level environment represents one's interpersonal proximal contexts. They include the structure and dynamics of the family; the values and social influences of peer groups, role models, and social networks; and the community and neighborhood in which youth live and interact, including schools, churches, health centers; and the physical environment.

Families are critical in the lives of youth in that they are responsible for material care, socializing children, and providing psychological supports of solidarity and cooperation, acceptance, comfort, and love (Barrow 2001). Parental expectations, evaluations, and encouragement or pressure also play a role in defining youth behaviors and outcomes (Feldman and Eliott 1997). Risk and protective factors are related to family dynamics and structure, with protective factors including: "connectedness," discipline (Hawkins et al. 1999), family resources (time, money, housing, and so forth), extended family (Burton, Allison, and Obeidallah 1995), two biological parents (Coleman 1988), parental presence (physical), family cohesion, and egalitarian gender roles and decisionmaking. "Connectedness" refers to a perception of closeness a young person has with a parent or family member; it is not based on doing things together but from a parent or family conveying psychological availability. Conversely, risk factors include low parental skills and education; scarce family resources; parental absence due to migration, job demands, or abandonment; abuse and violence in the household (physical, sexual, and emotional); parental mental health; parental substance abuse; and the presence of a nonbiological parent (World Bank 2001b, Furstenberg and Hughes 1995).

Social networks and supports are those friends, neighbors, friends of parents, and so forth on whom youth can rely to help cope with stresses and problems and decide on actions and behaviors. Likewise, peer groups—groups of the same age cohort or generation, groups with whom the youth "hangs out," or groups of similarly stereotyped individuals[5]—serve as an important source of values, directives, feedback, and social comparison (Feldman and Elliott 1997). Finally, role models are those persons that youth choose to emulate. Protective factors include having peers, social networks, and roles models that are positive and provide connectedness; peers and role models with prosocial norms; low-risk friends; and being treated fairly by peers. Conversely, risk factors include participation in deviant culture ("the bad boys"), perception of threat by peers, and prejudice.

The dynamics, structure, and organization of communities and neighborhoods help shape the lives, behaviors, and outcomes of adolescents. Their influences range from the provision of transportation systems, to the perceived degree of physical risk and safety, to community spirit and support. Churches, schools, sports and health centers, and other social organizations, which can provide a range of activities and supports to youth, are also part of the community and neighborhood infrastructure. Protective factors related to community and neighborhoods include well-functioning infrastructure, safe and secure spaces, trustworthy law enforcement officers, connectedness with organizations, and a clean physical environment. Conversely, risk factors associated with community include crime and violence; uncaring health center staff; the presence of alcohol and firearms; the lack of basic infrastructure, such as safe transportation; and corrupt local police officers.

Individual Factors

Individual risk and protective factors are those related to the physiological, cognitive, behavioral, social, and environmental systems. The physiological system is critical in that it determines physical health and growth; the cognitive system determines how individuals assimilate information, interpret it, and use it to make decisions; the behavioral system is key in that mortality and morbidity in

---

5. For example, typical stereotyped groups among students in the United States and Canada include "jocks, brains, loners, nerds," and so forth.

adolescence is mostly behaviorally based; the social system affects youth outcomes by establishing a social climate that favors specific behaviors; and social networks influence how adolescents deal with stressful events.

Some important risk factors at the individual level include having a physical or mental disability (Rutter 1993, Garmezy 1985, Werner 1982), aggressive behavior or rage, having a learning disability, and behaving in an ambivalent and unmotivated fashion. Protective factors at the individual level include spiritual belief (believing in a higher power beyond oneself), social skills, positive self-image and self-concept, self-confidence, having a positive and determined outlook, and being enterprising and hard-working. Perceived parental status is also a protective factor.

Risk-Taking Behaviors

Risk-taking behaviors are those actions taken by youth that hinder their personal development and successful integration into society (Barker and Fontes 1996). Such behaviors include not attending school, working in settings that are damaging to health and development (including working in illicit activities against one's will—e.g., prostitution), spending a large proportion of time on the streets (Barker and Fontes 1996), having unprotected or unsafe sex or engaging in sexual activities at an early age, being violent and participating in criminal behavior, and drug dealing and abusing drugs or other mind-altering substances. And given that societal systems affect at-risk behaviors, these can be gender differentiated.

Negative Youth Outcomes

Negative outcomes from risk-taking behaviors decrease the likelihood of having a healthy, happy, productive adult life. For example, adolescent pregnancy may predispose a person to low levels of education; school dropout or exit influences the attainment of human capital, which in turn affects job opportunities and earnings; youth unemployment affects a person's ability to gain experience, which in turn limits future job opportunities, earnings, and advancement; crime and violence lead to incarceration, which in turn affects one's ability to get a job, earn income, and marry, and so on.

It should be noted that negative outcomes can also be risk factors in and of themselves. For example, low human capital is a negative outcome of early school leaving, but it is also a risk factor because low levels of human capital predispose youth to other negative outcomes, such as unemployment, low earnings, and crime and violence. Similarly, sexual and physical abuse are a negative adult outcome, but they are also a risk factor in that they can predispose young people to mental health problems, risky sexual behavior, and crime and violence.

Adult Negative Outcomes

Low levels of education, poor work experience, low earnings, unemployment, poor physical and mental health, substance abuse, violence (including domestic violence), and unhealthy relationships with spouse, partner, friends and others are all adult outcomes that are influenced by negative youth outcomes.

3

NEGATIVE BEHAVIORS AND OUTCOMES OBSERVED AMONG CARIBBEAN YOUTH

Despite the Caribbean's historical, political, cultural, and linguistic diversity, the negative behaviors and outcomes observed among Caribbean youth are quite similar. These include early sexual initiation and pregnancy, HIV/AIDS, sexual and physical abuse, school leaving (dropout and exit), unemployment, crime and violence, substance abuse and drug dealing, and social exclusion. These outcomes and behaviors are discussed briefly in turn.

Early Sexual Initiation and Pregnancy

Early Sexual Initiation

The Caribbean region is characterized by a very early onset of sexual activity. Although other countries in the world (e.g., the United States) have a large proportion of sexually active adolescents, no other region in the world for which data are available have such an early age of sexual initiation (Blum 2002).[6] According to the nine-country CARICOM study, one-third of school-going young people were sexually active. Of these, more than half of boys and about a quarter of girls stated that the age at first intercourse was 10 years or younger, and almost two-thirds reported sexual initiation before the age of 13. In Jamaica, according to the reproductive health survey for 1997 (RHS-97), by age 11 to 12, about 20 percent of boys and girls in the general population have had sexual intercourse. In St. Lucia, almost 45 percent of sexually active adolescents engaged in first intercourse before the age of 10, according to the PAHO-funded St. Lucia 2000 adolescent health survey.[7] Early age of sexual initiation predisposes young people to early pregnancy, STIs, and HIV infection (Blum 2002).

Another issue particular to the Caribbean is that of forced intercourse. In the nine-country CARICOM study, of the one-third of adolescents who had had sexual intercourse, almost half

---

6. Sub-Saharan Africa is also characterized by early sexual initiation, but in contrast to the Africa region, most early sexual experiences in the Caribbean take place outside marriage.

7. The PAHO study, a school-based survey focused on age groups 10 to 19, surveyed 1,526 students from 29 primary and secondary schools island-wide.

reported that their first sexual experience had been forced. The proportion was high for both girls and boys: 48 percent and 32 percent, respectively. Although the problem of forced intercourse among girls is also problematic in other countries (such as the United States), the high incidence among boys is not common (Blum 2002).

Adolescent Pregnancy

Only four countries in the Americas have birth rates of more than 100 births per 1,000 women aged 15 to 19 years, and two of these are in the Caribbean (table 3-1). Antigua and Barbuda has

TABLE 3-1: FERTILITY RATES PER 1,000 WOMEN AGE 15–19*

Country	1996	1998	2000
Antigua & Barbuda	116.0	120.2	116.0
Argentina	66.3	62.6	58.8
Bahamas	62.5	62.9	57.8
Barbados	52.1	50.5	49.0
Belize	110.9	103.6	96.4
Canada	24.3	22.9	22.4
Chile	63.0	55.1	48.2
Colombia	58.6	55.6	52.6
Costa Rica	86.0	76.7	69.4
Dominica	28.9	27.4	25.8
Dominican Republic	110.4	105.9	101.4
Ecuador	82.9	76.8	70.7
El Salvador	115.5	110.2	104.8
Grenada	92.9	90.5	83.4
Guatemala	108.1	103.6	99.0
Guyana	27.3	25.7	24.0
Haiti	75.4	71.9	68.3
Honduras	127.2	118.2	109.3
Jamaica	66.2	53.5	40.9
Mexico	55.8	50.7	45.7
Panama	63.9	55.9	48.0
Peru	67.8	61.3	54.7
St. Kitts & Nevis	77.2	70.5	63.8
Saint Lucia	65.9	58.5	51.1
St. Vincent and the Grenadines	77.2	46.4	34.6
Suriname	36.9	34.5	32.0
Trinidad & Tobago	20.8	18.7	16.7
United States	55.6	61.5	58.2
Uruguay	52.0	51.1	50.2
Venezuela	74.6	65.0	55.3

Source: www.paho.org/English/SHA/coredata
* The ratio between the number of live births born to mothers aged 15 to 19 years during a given year and the mid-year female population 15 to 19 years of age, usually multiplied by 1,000.

the highest adolescent pregnancy rates in the Americas, followed by Honduras, El Salvador, and the Dominican Republic. But rates vary widely in the Caribbean. At the other end of the spectrum, Trinidad and Tobago has the lowest rate in the Americas (16.7 per 1,000 women aged 15 to 19). Only seven countries in the Americas have rates lower than 45 births per 1,000 women aged 15 to 19 years, and six of these are in the Caribbean (Trinidad and Tobago, Guyana, Dominica, Suriname, St. Vincent and the Grenadines, and Jamaica). Belize and Grenada have fairly high rates of teen pregnancy (96.4 and 83.4, respectively), and the other five countries fall somewhere in the middle (Haiti, St. Kitts and Nevis, the Bahamas, Barbados, and St. Lucia). In terms of pregnancies, the CARICOM survey revealed that about 10 percent of school-going adolescents had been pregnant or had gotten someone regnant (7 percent in the case of girls and 12 percent in the case of boys). The proportion is probably higher among school leavers.

Despite high levels of sexual activity among adolescents, contraceptive use remains low. Only a quarter of CARICOM's school-going, sexually active sample were using some form of birth control, and only slightly more worry about getting pregnant or causing a pregnancy. In Jamaica, more than 40 percent of sexually active adolescent girls reported that they had not used, a contraceptive at last intercourse, and 87 percent of teenage pregnancies had not been planned (World Bank 2001b).

Risky Sexual Behavior and HIV/AIDS

After Sub-Saharan Africa, the Caribbean region currently has the highest HIV/AIDS prevalence rate in the world—and data suggest that for one-third of all new cases, the disease was contracted when the individual was aged 15 to 24 years.[8] Out of the 12 countries with the highest HIV prevalence in the Latin America and the Caribbean (LAC) Region, nine are from the Caribbean (World Bank 2000a). HIV/AIDS has reached epidemic proportions in countries such as Haiti, the Bahamas, and Guyana. Jamaica and Trinidad and Tobago have concentrated HIV/AIDS epidemics.[9] About 83 percent of AIDS cases are diagnosed in people between the ages of 15 and 54; one-third of all new cases are in the 25- to 34-year-old age group (see table 3-2). Given an estimated 8- to 10-year incubation period, about one-third of those who have new AIDS cases contracted the disease when they were 15 to 24 years old.

The high incidence of HIV among youth has been linked to early sexual initiation and low condom use among young people. According to the nine-country CARICOM study of school-attending adolescents, almost half (47 percent) of sexually active youth reported not using a condom. The majority of St. Lucia at-risk youth interviewed for the qualitative study indicated that they were worried about HIV/AIDS—however, the use and knowledge of contraception was low. In Jamaica, the level of knowledge about sexuality and contraception is reportedly high among adolescents, but it does not translate into preventive behavior, according to the RHS-97 (World Bank 2001b).

Physical and Sexual Abuse
Physical Abuse
Many of the young people surveyed in the nine-country CARICOM study report a history of abuse in their lives. About one-sixth state that they have been physically abused, with most of the abuse being attributed to an adult in their home. Evidence from Jamaica, Barbados, and Dominica suggests that parents' use of harsh disciplinary action on children is common. A quantitative study on

---

8. Among women, the majority of cases are in the 25- to 29-year-old age bracket, followed by the 30- to 34-year-old age group; among men, the majority of cases are in the 30 to 34 and 25 to 29 age cohort (PAHO/WHO 1998, cited in World Bank 2000a).

9. According to World Bank (2000a), a generalized epidemic means that HIV has spread far beyond the original subpopulations with high-risk behavior (defined as engaging in unprotected sexual intercourse with many partners or sharing unsterilized needles or other injecting equipment); a concentrated epidemic means that HIV/AIDS is still primarily affecting population groups practicing high-risk behaviors (among whom infection rates exceed 5 percent) but are set to spread more widely in the rest of the population.

TABLE 3-2: REPORTED CASES OF AIDS BY AGE GROUP, CARIBBEAN REGION

Age group	<1990	1990	1991	1992	1993	1994	1995	1996	1997	1998	1999	2000	1982–2000	%
<1	78	21	29	34	37	47	33	39	44	32	43	32	469	3
1–4	47	14	13	25	17	28	36	69	41	49	63	61	463	3
5–14	5	6	4	6	7	12	14	18	11	8	22	23	136	1
15–19	34	13	14	11	20	25	21	43	21	23	49	24	298	2
20–24	186	74	80	87	70	88	128	111	100	108	166	109	1,307	8
25–29	329	110	120	165	195	209	234	242	244	218	314	240	2,620	15
30–34	315	120	152	182	192	210	312	299	286	360	389	280	3,097	18
35–39	195	87	132	159	201	269	256	275	294	295	368	293	2,824	16
40–44	140	57	96	93	124	124	192	222	220	209	292	220	1,989	12
45–49	89	46	69	65	85	123	129	140	93	150	167	204	1,360	8
50–54	71	20	50	34	67	54	87	107	90	103	122	111	916	5
55–59	43	22	23	35	33	59	41	69	67	81	87	75	635	4
>60	48	22	33	38	44	35	73	78	59	80	77	80	667	4
Unknown	121	50	49	89	25	15	26	16	33	30	27	54	535	3
Total (all ages)	1,701	662	864	1,023	1,117	1,298	1,582	1,728	1,603	1,746	2,186	1,806	17,316	100

Source: Quarterly AIDS surveillance reports submitted to CAREC's Epidemiology Division by CAREC member countries.

sexual decisionmaking in Jamaica revealed that 50 percent of all respondents had reportedly been severely punished as children (beaten, punched, pinched, or hit with a heavy object [Wyatt et al. 1993, cited in Le Franc 2001]). Another study carried out in Jamaica, Barbados, and Dominica suggested similar harsh disciplinary patterns, with the physical punishment of boys being particularly severe (Le Franc 2001). Making boys tough and controlling boys is typically the justification for the harsher punishment of the male child.

Cultural norms sanction the practice of corporal punishment to discipline children. Schools, for example, continue to use corporal punishment to impose discipline (Rock 2001, Meeks-Gardener 2001). A study of 29 schools in primary and all-ages schools in Jamaica showed that in 27 of the 29 schools, 87 percent of teachers and children reported that beatings occurred as an act of punishment, with teachers using a strap, belt, or ruler (Meeks-Gardener 2001). Boys tend to be treated more harshly than girls within the school environment (Rock 2001). Corporal punishment is also used widely by parents to teach their children to be compliant in countries such as Barbados (Rock 2001) and Jamaica (World Bank 2001b).

Sexual Abuse

Similarly, many of the young people surveyed in the nine-country CARICOM study report a history of sexual abuse in their lives. One-tenth report having been abused sexually, most frequently by adults outside the home or other teens, but many report abuse by adults in the home and siblings. There is remarkably little gender difference between males (9.1 percent) and females (10.5 percent) reporting sexual abuse. About one in eight reports that they worry they will be sexually abused.

A 1993 study in Jamaica suggests a certain "normalcy" attached to the act of child sexual abuse (Rock 2001). The study, however, challenges popular beliefs about the abuse of children by stepfathers and mothers' boyfriends,[10] instead finding that a greater level of abuse was taking place in two-parent households or in households where the relatives of the father were raising the child. Rock's more recent (2001) study of child abuse in Barbados supports this assertion. According to study findings, parents were reportedly the main perpetrators of child abuse in all categories except sexual abuse: Mothers made up the majority of perpetrators of physical abuse (49.4 percent), nonfamily members made up the majority of sexual offenders of children (55.5 percent),[11] and mothers made up the majority of those who neglect their children (68.0 percent). Rock also found that the reported cases of child abuse and neglect were increasing in Barbados.[12]

School Leaving

As with other indicators, the number of out-of-school youth varies significantly across Caribbean countries. According to data compiled by the CYP, the proportion of youth whose highest level of education is primary school is as high as 58 percent in Dominica, 54 percent in Belize, and 53 percent in St. Vincent and the Grenadines (Danns, Henry, and LaFleur 1997). In Jamaica in 1999, 2.5 percent of 12-to 14-year-olds were not in school, but by the age of 15 to 16 years, the proportion of school leavers was almost 17 percent, which reflects a significant dropout rate at the secondary education level (Samms-Vaughan 2001). Secondary enrollment rates also remain low in the Dominican Republic. In 1998, net secondary enrollment was 17 percent for boys and 36 percent for girls; in urban areas, the rates were 40 percent for boys and 47 percent for girls (World Bank

---

10. Indeed, according to perceptions of St. Lucia key informants of this study, the preponderance of loosely attached males within most single-parent families leads to a high level of sexual abuse of female adolescents within the home setting. It is so commonly perceived that stepfathers are acting as sexual predators on female youth that in 2001, a calypso was written on this social problem.

11. The data indicated that 19.8 percent of sexual offenders were the children's fathers, 13.8 percent were the stepfathers, and 10.9 percent were other family members.

12. A total of 763 cases were referred to the Child Care Board between April 1989 and March 1990; from April to March 1997–98, the cases reported were 1,132, and 1,113 from April to March 1998–99 (Rock 2001). Underreporting of cases is suspected, however, given that reporting is not mandatory.

2001b). Not surprisingly, net enrollment rates are significantly higher among the nonpoor than the poor (World Bank 2001b). Also, the proportion of boys who do not attend secondary school is similar for the nonpoor and the poor after controlling for wealth variables.

Across the Caribbean, more boys than girls tend to fall behind and leave school. In the case of Jamaica, in 1996–97 and 1999–2000, a slightly higher proportion of boys than girls were enrolled at the early childhood and primary school levels; at grades 7 to 9, females accounted for just over 50 percent of enrollment; and at grades 10 to 11, the gender gap widened in favor of females, with a percentage gap of 8.8 and 5.2 between male and female enrollment in 1996–97 and 1999–2000, respectively. In St. Vincent and the Grenadines, for the 1991–92 school year, the ratio of female to male students was nearly 1.5 to 1 (Barker 1995). And gender gaps in grade repetition and dropout in the Dominican Republic are among the widest in Latin America (World Bank 2001b).[13]

Unemployment

As in other parts of the world, unemployment in the Caribbean is primarily a youth phenomenon (see tables 3-3 and 3-4). Across countries in the Caribbean and elsewhere, youth unemployment rates—that is, the number of 15- to 24-year-olds looking for work as a proportion of the sum of 15- to 24-year-olds that are either working or looking for work—are double to quadruple the adult rates. International comparisons, however, indicate that some Caribbean countries have particularly high youth unemployment rates. According to the *World Development Indicators,* from 1996 to 1998, St. Lucia had the highest rate in the Americas and the Caribbean, followed by Jamaica (among those countries for which data were available).[14] Caribbean-wide data indicate

TABLE 3-3: YOUTH AND ADULT UNEMPLOYMENT IN THE CARIBBEAN									
		Youth (15–24 years) unemployment (%)			Adult unemployment (%)			Youth as share of unemployed (%)		
Country	Year	All	Male	Female	All	Male	Female	All	Male	Female
Antigua and Barbuda	1991	13.0	13.1	12.8	4.2	4.0	4.4	47.0	47.5	46.0
Anguilla	1992	13.7	14.1	13.0	4.0	4.0	3.9	55.1	56.3	52.9
Barbados	1999	17.9	15.2	20.9	7.4	5.2	9.6	36.6	41.8	33.3
Belize	1999	18.4	13.4	25.8	8.2	6.1	12.1	50.8	47.7	53.5
Dominica	1997	28.1	28.9	26.7	14.4	15.3	12.6	40.9	39.5	43.8
Grenada	1998	23.9	21.1	28.2	9.2	5.3	13.5	49.0	59.8	43.8
Guyana	1992	21.1	17.2	27.7	5.2	3.2	8.8	66.9	72.0	62.3
Jamaica	1999	25.4	19.1	31.8	8.9	5.4	12.8	52.6	57.2	50.1
St. Lucia	1998	30.6	27.7	34.0	12.5	9.9	15.4	50.0	54.2	46.4
St. Vincent and the Grenadines	1991	26.7	24.7	30.0	11.2	10.8	11.9	55.3	54.2	57.1
Trinidad and Tobago	1999	20.2	17.9	23.6	8.8	7.2	11.2	42.8	44.1	41.6

Source: ILO 1999.

---

13. Completion rates for boys from the richest 20 percent of households are higher than for girls, and completion rates for girls from poorer households are higher than for boys. This suggests that poor boys are left behind or are pressed to drop out of school to provide income support to the family, whereas traditional domestic work typically carried out by poor girls is more compatible with schooling.

14. See http://www.worldbank.org/data. Countries for which data were available included the Bahamas, Barbados, Brazil, Canada, Chile, Colombia, Costa Rica, Ecuador, Honduras, Jamaica, Mexico, Panama, St. Lucia, Suriname, the United States, Uruguay, and Venezuela. Following St. Lucia and Jamaica, Panama, Trinidad and Tobago, and Barbados had the highest rates, in that order.

TABLE 3-4: UNEMPLOYMENT LEVELS IN THE DOMINICAN REPUBLIC BY AGE GROUP, URBAN OR RURAL RESIDENCE, AND SEX

								Youth relative to total	
Urban									
	15–19	20–24	25–34	35–44	45–54	55–70	Total	(15–19)	(20–24)
Male	29.4	19.6	8.4	5.0	5.2	5.8	11.2	2.63	1.75
Female	53.1	40.5	22.2	17.8	14.4	13.8	25.3	2.10	1.6
Rural								Youth relative to total	
	15–19	20–24	25–34	35–44	45–54	55–70	Total	(15–19)	(20–24)
Male	17.2	9.0	5.0	1.1	1.1	6.1	6.2	1.54	0.80
Female	49.8	33.9	23.2	19.4	14	8.9	24.4	1.97	1.34

Source: World Bank (2001b) based on *Encuesta Nacional de Gastos e Ingresos del Hogar*, 1998.

St. Lucia, followed by Dominica, St. Vincent and the Grenadines, and Jamaica have the highest youth unemployment rates (see table 3-3).

In those Caribbean countries where all unemployment is high, many youth are "discouraged workers," meaning that they would like to work but do not even bother looking for a job because they know that they will not find it. Thus, youth unemployment is likely to be underestimated in high unemployment economies. Nonetheless, youth in the Caribbean make up 20 to 30 percent of the labor force but represent 40 to 60 percent of the unemployed (with the exception of Barbados).

Youth unemployment rates are higher for females than males, although their proportion of the total unemployed labor force tends to be less (see tables 3-4 and 3-5). This means that fewer young women than young men are in the labor force, but within their respective gender groups, a larger share of young females is unemployed. In the English-speaking Caribbean, the gender differential is greatest in Belize, followed by the Bahamas, Jamaica, and Guyana. Gender differentials in the Dominican Republic are even greater, with rates for young rural women aged 20 to 24 years being almost triple those of rates for young rural men. Last, as the Dominican Republic data indicate (table 3-5) unemployment is primarily an urban problem, and male urban youth have the highest share of total unemployment (concentration factor of 2.63).

Crime and Violence
Based on homicide rates, the LAC Region as a whole is the most violent region in the world. At 22.9 per 100,000 people in 1990, homicide rates for the Caribbean are almost double the world average of 10.7 per 100,000[15]—and as in the rest of the LAC Region, available data indicate that homicide victims and perpetrators are disproportionately young men.[16] Within the Caribbean, Jamaica's homicide rates are the highest (35 homicides per 100,000) and levels for the Dominican Republic and Trinidad and Tobago exceed the world average (11.7 and 12.6 homicides per 100,000, respectively) (Ayres 1998). Violence also appears to be mounting in the larger islands; for example, it increased sixfold in Trinidad and Tobago from the early 1980s to the early 1990s. Violent crimes tend to be geographically concentrated in poor urban communities (Ayres 1998), with Kingston, Jamaica, reportedly having one of the highest murder rates in the world.[17]

---

15. Rates are for 1990, which was the last year for which subregional Caribbean data were available.
16. Homicide victims and perpetrators in the Americas are disproportionately men aged 15 to 24 years (PAHO 1993, cited in Barker 1998).
17. *Sunday Gleaner,* October 17, 1998.

TABLE 3-5: PROSECUTED CRIME IN JAMAICA BY AGE GROUP, 1998		
Offense	Ages 17 to –25, as share of all crimes (%)	Ages 17 29, as share of all crimes (%)
Murder	47.8	84.8
Manslaughter	44.4	80.0
Felonious wounding	32.1	64.1
Sex offenses	38.9	74.4
Burglary	41.7	64.1
Robbery	55.1	74.6
Breach of firearms act	64.0	81.3
Shooting with intent	100.0	100.0
Larceny	67.4	84.7
Arson	33.3	33.3
Forgery	49.3	77.5
Unlawful possession	83.3	100.0
Breach of drug laws	62.1	85.3
Other offenses	60.9	84.2
All crimes	55.7	79.6

Source: Pantin 2000.

Department of Corrections data for Jamaica show that young people (aged 17 to 30) commit most offenses, with youth (aged 15 to 24) contributing significantly to crime and violence (table 3-5). Youth aged 17 to 25 commit 56 percent of all crimes, almost 50 percent of murders, 44 percent of manslaughters, and 42 percent of burglaries. Available information for Jamaica indicates that perpetrators of crime tend to be young men. In 2000, 20- to 25-year-old males were the principal offenders in all types of major crimes in Jamaica and accounted for 37 percent of all murders committed in that year, according to the Planning Institute of Jamaica (PIOJ) *Economic and Social Survey of Jamaica* (1999)

Young men also tend to be the main victims of homicides. Based on 1990 data, a 1993 Commission on Youth in Barbados found that youth were much more likely to die from homicide and purposefully inflicted injuries than any other age group. Young people made up nearly two-thirds of those found guilty of crimes; males were four times more likely than females to be found guilty of a crime, with the sex differential having increased every year since 1960 (Braithwaite 1993, cited in Pantin 2000). In Jamaica, among patients seen in emergency units of public hospitals with trauma and injuries related to acts of violence in 2000, the highest proportion of patients were 20- to 29-year-olds (31.6 percent), followed by 30- to 39-year-olds (29.8 percent) and 10- to 19-year-olds (22.3 percent) (PIOJ, based on Ministry of Health data, cited in World Bank 2001b).[18]

---

18. It is important to note that whereas young people are more likely to be victims of violence, most Caribbean countries tend to have youthful populations, thus explaining the concentration of homicides among youth. Comparing trends of homicide victims for the United States and Trinidad and Tobago, for example, shows that as the population ages in Trinidad and Tobago, the risk of dying by homicide decreases. This is not the case in the United States, where the share of homicide victims tends to be concentrated among youth despite an aging population.

The nine-country CARICOM study of school-age youth, as well as the qualitative information from the Dominican Republic, confirms the presence of violence in the lives of youth. One-fifth of males in the CARICOM survey had carried weapons to school in the previous 30 days of the survey, and nearly as many had been in a fight using weapons. Also, the gang violence rate is high, with one in five school-going boys and one in eight school-going girls indicating that they had at some time belonged to a gang. Out-of-school youth interviewed in the Dominican Republic substantiate the presence of gangs and violence in their communities. Youth tend to join criminal and drug-dealing gangs to compensate for lack of formal employment opportunities or as a strategy for confronting the violence in their communities. Gangs and political parties were the organizations with whom youth mostly identified.

Rage is apparently a common sentiment among Caribbean youth, with more than 40 percent of teenagers reporting such emotions, according to the CARICOM survey of school-going youth. Two out of five report that sometimes or most of the time they think about hurting or killing someone else, and almost 5 percent report that they almost always think about hurting or killing others. Males consistently report rage significantly more often than their female counterparts in every age group of teens. About one in eight of youth surveyed have tried to kill themselves, with no appreciable differences between males and females or different age groups.

Substance Abuse and Drug Dealing

According to a United Nations International Drug Control Programme (UNDCP)–funded study, drug and substance abuse and youth involvement in drug dealing are significant problems facing at-risk youth in the Caribbean (Barker 1995). Although data and information are scanty, the study—which involved St. Vincent and the Grenadines, Trinidad and Tobago, St. Martin and Jamaica—summarized the situation as follows:

> Both among in-school and out-of-school youth, there is a widespread social acceptance of alcohol and marijuana in the Caribbean. Youth interviewed in focus group discussions tended to rank drugs according to their acceptability, with alcohol being the most heavily used and accepted, marijuana second and cocaine last. Both marijuana and alcohol were seen as socially acceptable, while cocaine and crack were seen as more dangerous and more extreme in their side effects and their implications.

The study also found that the group most at risk of substance abuse and involvement in drug dealing were out-of-school youth aged 13 to 19, particularly male youth. By country examined, the study revealed the following:

- *St. Vincent and the Grenadines:* Statistics from 1990 to 1994 found that about 12 to 16 percent of all inmates had been imprisoned for drug-related charges; other theft and larceny charges are also likely to be drug related. The majority of the inmates were 16- to 30-year-olds. Although there are no statistics on substance abuse among out-of-school youth, a 1993 survey of 1,428 students in St. Vincent and the Grenadines (representing 81 percent of 11- to 16-year-olds) found that alcohol was the most widely used substance, with 89.9 percent saying they had used alcohol, and 34 percent had used in the past 30 days. Only 11.5 percent reported they had used marijuana, and fewer than 1 percent had ever used cocaine.
- *Trinidad and Tobago:* Recent studies have found fairly high rates of substance use among in-school youth, as well as widespread access. In general, alcohol and marijuana are the most widely accepted and the most widely available. One 1992 study of youth in primary and secondary schools found that 14 percent of youth in primary schools said that marijuana was easy to obtain, and 12 percent said the same for cocaine. At the secondary level, 38 percent said marijuana was easy to obtain, and 13 percent said cocaine was easy to obtain. In terms of substance abuse in schools, various studies carried out between 1985 and 1988 found that among 11- to 19-year-olds, between 80.4 percent and 91.1 percent

had used alcohol, between 6.3 percent and 10.6 percent had used marijuana, and between 1.1 percent and 3.3 percent had used cocaine.

■ *Jamaica:* Although no data were available, anecdotal evidence points to a major problem in substance abuse and drug dealing among out-of-school youth in Jamaica. The most recent survey on drug use among in-school youth was carried out by the Jamaican government in 1997, and it found that 71 percent had used alcohol, 27 percent had smoked ganja (marijuana), and 2 percent had tried cocaine. Higher percentages appear to drink marijuana brewed as tea. Various qualitative studies have concluded that young out-of-school males from low-income families are the group most likely to use drugs. Similarly, anecdotal evidence suggests that many youth are involved in drug trafficking and drug dealing. Some youth report that drug dealers are currently role models for many youth, especially males.

Both at-risk and control youth groups in the St. Lucia qualitative study suggested that alcohol use was widespread and in most cases began in the early to preteen years. According to the 2000 PAHO adolescent health study for St. Lucia, 63.3 percent of in-school teens surveyed had taken an alcoholic drink in the year preceding the study, and almost 10 percent drank alcohol on a monthly or more frequent basis.[19]

Social Exclusion

Numerous authors and researchers have described or referred to Caribbean youth and at-risk youth as feeling powerless and excluded from the mainstream of Caribbean societies (Danns, Henry, and LaFleur 1997; James-Bryant 1992; Deosaran 1992; Lewis 1995; West Indian Commission 1992; Barker 1995). This is not surprising, given that the social integration of youth involves the insertion into the workforce and political, social, and cultural life, as well as a smooth transition from dependence on the family to independence (Morales 2001). In the case of many Caribbean nations—with their inequality of educational opportunity, high levels of youth unemployment, and precarious employment—many youth face extreme difficulties in completing this passage, which is a key component of future healthy adult life and well-being (Danns, Henry, and LaFleur 1997).

According to the St. Lucia qualitative data, a large number of at-risk youth feel excluded from decision making in the development of the country and even from their own communities. In addition, at-risk youth—especially males from ghettos—are branded and socially excluded because of the communities in which they reside, further promoting their isolation. Qualitative data collected among at-risk youth in the Dominican Republic suggest similar patterns. Interviews there revealed the following:

This youth's social life takes place in an atmosphere that lacks such minimum services such as electricity, water, adequate homes, clubs, sports facilities, libraries, health services. While neighborhoods have schools, these are few and do not meet demand. Thus the social life of youth is extremely deficient.

Even when community-based organizations existed in their neighborhoods, the youngsters were excluded. For example, in rural areas, young women who are pregnant or have children, cannot access cultural community groups that offer technical education because these groups are targeted to young female virgins with no sexual experience.

The strongest organizations (drug dealers and gangs) dominate the environment in many poor communities. They are the ones that set the rules of the game in these settlements.

---

19. The 2000 PAHO-funded St. Lucia adolescent health survey surveyed 1,526 students from 29 primary and secondary schools island-wide.

Youth played an active role in the birth of politically independent Caribbean (Lewis 1995), but disillusion among youth followed.[20] Postcolonial Caribbean youth have found themselves in societies in which "the rhetoric of self-reliance, of new visions for youth, of education as a vehicle for democracy, of youth entrepreneurship, all these promises did not materialize in viable amounts" (Deosaran 1992). Youth had come to realize that they were living in a political culture where "nepotism crowns geriatric politics" (Deosaran 1992). Indeed young people found that " in large measure, the politics of colonialism have given way to a political independence which provides its own entrenched elites, leaving a blockade against change and youthful succession" (Deosaran 1992).

Disillusion and distrust appear to have led to indifference. According to Barker (1995), many youth—particularly at-risk youth—do not use the programs set up for them by government and non-governmental organizations (NGOs) because these youth have lost trust in institutions. Dominican Republic informants suggest that youth indifference is a major problem among those faced with the most risk factors. According to these sources, attracting youth to community organizations is increasingly difficult because of disinterest among youth. Similarly, St. Lucian at-risk urban youth who were interviewed voiced disinterest in and negativity toward community activities. The data indicate that, as in other parts of the world, those youth who most need special services and supports are those youth most reluctant or least likely to use these services.

---

20. "Throughout the Caribbean during the 1930s it was the bulk of the young people who were among the chief architects of the labour revolts of that time" (Lewis 1995, 9). The social unrest of the 1930s not only gave birth to the labor movement in the Caribbean but also provided the political leadership for the independence movements in the region. In the 1970s, many young people—particularly students—across the region supported the black power movement in an attempt to realize Bob Marley's call to emancipate black people from mental slavery and as a response to the residue of racism still embedded in the social structures of the region. Young people played an active role in both the attempted coup in Trinidad and Tobago in 1990 and the Grenadian revolution in 1979.

4

SOURCES OF POSITIVE AND NEGATIVE YOUTH OUTCOMES

This chapter identifies primary risk and protective factors associated with youth development in the Caribbean, which may be thought of as policy intervention points. Although the problems facing youth in the Caribbean are well known and often discussed, the causes behind the observed risk-taking behavior and negative youth outcomes remain a mystery. A better understanding of those factors associated with risk-taking behaviors is necessary for appropriate program design and policy.

The quantitative data in this chapter provide an estimate of the correlation between risk or protective factors and risk-taking youth behavior or outcomes, and the qualitative data are used to explain the quantitative findings and suggest causality. Because of the cross-sectional nature of the quantitative data, it is not possible to identify a particular risk factor as the cause of an observed behavior or if other unobservable characteristics are responsible for the correlation. For example, statistics show that youth who attend religious services are also those who have a lower tendency for substance abuse. This finding does not allow one to deduce that religious service attendance leads to lower substance abuse or that lower substance abuse leads to religious service attendance. The causation may go in either direction, or a completely different factor may be affecting both behaviors, causing the observed correlation, such as a supportive family structure that leads to both lower substance abuse and religious service attendance. Because causal relationships cannot be determined by the quantitative data, the qualitative data are exploited, where appropriate, to suggest causal relationships.

The most pertinent risk and protective factors in each of the categories in figure 2-1 are discussed here. Although each category of risk or protective factor is discussed independently, it is important to note that there is a high degree of interconnectedness among the risk or protective categories. Most of the supporting evidence in this chapter is drawn from three sources: Blum (2002); Luther, St. Ville, and Hasbún (2002); and Barker (1995). The first source is a background paper prepared for this study that uses data collected from schoolchildren in nine CARICOM countries to examine the connection among family, school, community, self, and risk-taking behaviors.[21] The paper by Luther, St. Ville, and Hasbún (2002), which was also prepared specifically for this study, reports findings from focus groups and youth experts in St. Lucia and the Dominican Republic who discussed the factors that lead to the challenges facing youth today. Finally, Barker's study (1995), which was prepared for the U.N., reports discussions with focus groups and youth experts about the use and sale of drugs in St. Martin, Jamaica, St. Vincent and the Grenadines, and Trinidad and Tobago. The methodology used in the background papers prepared for this report is discussed in appendix 2; the methodology for Barker (1995) can be found in the source. The terminology used in this chapter is given in appendix 2.

Individual

Youth who display low self-esteem, rage, ambivalence, or hopelessness are also those who are exposed to risk factors and engage in risk-taking behaviors. These negative dispositions may be biological, the propensity for the behavior may be biological but is triggered by the environment, or they may be purely learned. Regardless of whether these are truly exogenous feelings or a result of the environment, they are correlated with unfavorable activities.

Self-esteem: A positive self-image is a fundamental factor in protecting youth from consuming drugs or alcohol, engaging in violence, or initiating sexual activity. Risk factors correlated with low self-esteem among Caribbean youth are primarily found in the household: maternal emotional abandonment,[22] an absence of parental nurturing (connectedness), unskilled parents, and sexual abuse in the household that is known and accepted by other adults. Additionally, the exclusionary nature of the school system—both in expelling children from school who do not pass the entrance exams and the social ranking in secondary schools by the color of uniform worn[23]—and poverty that includes coming from the "wrong" neighborhood were identified by St. Lucian youth as negative influences on self-esteem.

Rage: Feelings of rage are prevalent among youth who use tobacco, alcohol, and drugs; undertake violent activity; and prematurely engage in sexual activity.[24] Holding all else constant, fewer than 10 percent of school-going boys and 5 percent of school-going girls who do not feel rage smoke tobacco or consume alcohol, and fewer than 20 percent use drugs. Conversely, among those school-going youth who do express feelings of rage, the use of tobacco and alcohol doubles for boys and triples for girls, and drug use approaches 30 percent (figures 4-1 and 4-2). Although the data do not allow us to test for causality, it is likely that tobacco use is a result of rage rather than a cause of it.

Similar increases are seen with violence and sexual experience, where 22 percent of boys and 9 percent of girls who are happy engage in violence compared with 70 percent of boys and 40 percent of girls who feel rage. Sexual experience, which is a high 35 percent for boys and 13 percent for girls who attend school, nearly doubles with male rage and increases 2.5 times for girls who feel rage. When controlling for age, these same propensities emerge. With respect to suicide, feelings of rage increase suicide thoughts or attempts by 14.6 percent, especially among boys (Blum 2002).

The sources of rage may include family, institutions, and limited economic opportunities. An aggressive family is a key correlate with rage, and connectedness with parents is a key correlated

---

21. Because of an agreement with the participating countries, country-by-country results cannot be presented. However, able A1.1 found in appendix 1 shows that the regression results are very similar across countries, allowing us to generalize across the sample countries.

22. Maternal emotional abandonment alludes to mothers giving up on their children and holding them responsible for their own failings, thus contributing to low self-esteem (Luther, St. Ville, and Hasbun 2002).

23. In many countries, youth are assigned to secondary schools based on their performance of the Common Entrance Exams. Each school has its own uniform, thus attendance at a more prestigious secondary school is clearly signalled by the uniform worn by the young person, which also speaks loudly about his or her ranking on the CEEs.

24. Nearly 40 percent of girls and 47 percent of boys in the English-speaking Caribbean countries think about hurting or killing someone—a proxy for rage. This propensity increases and deepens with age (Blum 2002). The estimated odds ratio between rage and risky behaviors is significant at the 1 percent level as follows: violence (2.44–3.23, higher for boys), sexual initiation (1.7–1.8), and substance abuse (1.24–1.63 for ages 13 to 15 and 16 to 18) (Blum 2002).

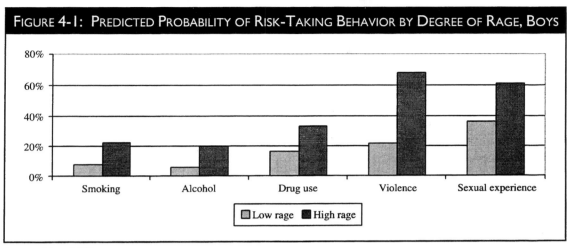

FIGURE 4-1: PREDICTED PROBABILITY OF RISK-TAKING BEHAVIOR BY DEGREE OF RAGE, BOYS

Source: Blum 2002.

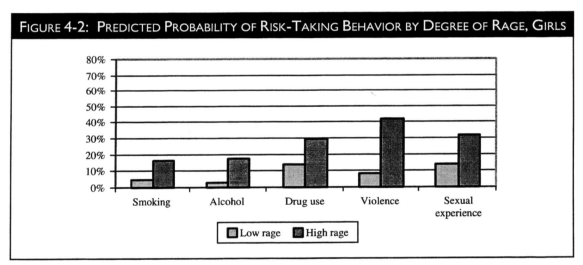

FIGURE 4-2: PREDICTED PROBABILITY OF RISK-TAKING BEHAVIOR BY DEGREE OF RAGE, GIRLS

Source: Blum 2002.

protective factor.[25] More than half of school-going youth who feel rage have been physically or sexually abused by family members, and 38 percent of those who feel rage have not suffered abuse (table 4-1). Those who feel connected to their families are only half as likely to feel rage, especially among girls (Blum 2002). This is constant across age.

Connectedness to other adults and religious institutions also is associated with lower rage, but the school and justice systems are correlated with higher levels of rage. Qualitative evidence suggests that these institutions create rage. For example, young people in St. Lucia report that expulsion from school as a result of failing entrance exams or wearing the uniform of a less prestigious school instills anger toward the system in young people. This is exacerbated in poor areas, where the interviewed youth (in the Dominican Republic and St. Lucia) feel that police authorities are

25. The estimated odds ratio when regressing the probability of feeling rage on the parental abuse variable ranges from 1.27 to 1.53, with a higher value for younger children (ages 10 to 12). This is significant at the 1 percent level. The family connectedness estimate ranges from 0.44 to 0.51, again with the largest effects for the youngest children (Blum 2002).

TABLE 4-1: THE RELATIONSHIP BETWEEN EXPERIENCING ABUSE AND EMOTIONAL DISTRESS				
Emotional distress[a]	No abuse (%)	Physical abuse (%)	Sexual abuse (%)	Both (%)
Depression (50.4%)	45.7	65.4	61.9	69.7
Rage (40.1%)	37.8	54.7	53.5	51.2
Suicide attempt (12.1%)	9.1	20.1	23.1	28.9

a. Percent of total sample reporting.

Source: PAHO Adolescent Health Survey 2000.

aggressive and prejudiced. Finally, the lack of job opportunities in a stagnant economy was identified as a source of youth anger (Barker 1995; Luther, St. Ville, and Hasbún 2002).

Ambivalence: A key observation of those who work with youth is that young people are less willing to be proactive in support of the public good, instead preferring to put their energies toward personal needs. Many youth programs depend on the participation of young people, who were key to political struggles in the 1970s (Williams 2002, Alexis 2000) and to putting youth on the agenda in the 1980s (Williams 2002, National Youth Council—St. Lucia). Increased individualism and consumerism, which both youth experts and young people themselves trace to U.S. media images and inequality that is highlighted by the tourist and drug trades, teach young people to put energies into themselves (Barker 1995). When voluntary community action takes place, the motivations are often personal, rather than collective. This is clearly expressed by a young man in the Dominican Republic who said, "We fight so that they can fix our streets because you buy a pair of new sneakers and this street with all the dirt damages them." (Luther, St. Ville, and Hasbún 2002).

Hopelessness: Ambivalence may be a reaction to the hopelessness felt by young people who believe that they have no chance for happy, productive lives because the institutional and economic systems do not offer any chances for advancement (Barker 1995). In particular, youth reported that corruption in public institutions leads to inefficient use of resources and a failure of the state to respond to their needs, whether medical, security, educational, or social protection. Additionally, the exclusionary nature of the school system denies many children the opportunity for secondary or college-level education, which youth identify as a key input to finding good jobs in the future. Even those who do obtain education will enter a highly competitive job market where jobs are scarce and well-paying jobs are even more difficult to find.

Microenvironment

The microenvironment—those institutions and influences that the young person confronts daily—are a source of both risk and protective factors, as discussed in chapter 2. The microfactors differ from the macrofactors in that the former are those influences that are confronted on a very close, personal level, and the latter are shared across all youth on a national level. In the context of the Caribbean, the research reveals the importance, first and foremost, of the family and the high correlation between familial protective factors and positive youth behaviors, on the one hand, and familial risk factors and youth risk-taking behaviors, on the other hand. Other important microenvironmental forces are peers, roles models, social networks, and the community or neighborhood.

Family

Familial behavior is both the strongest protective factor and a risk factor in youth development. It is a protective factor in that family connectedness (Resnick and Hojat, 1997; Blum and Rinehart 1997), appropriate levels of parental discipline (Barker 1995), moral guidance, protection from dangers in the adult world, and economic support allow young people to acquire personal and social skills while young (Luther, St. Ville, and Hasbun 2002). However, parental displays of negative behaviors (drug use, alcohol abuse, violence, low commitment to family); physical, sexual, and emotional abuse by family members or within the home; and the absence of parental guidance and support

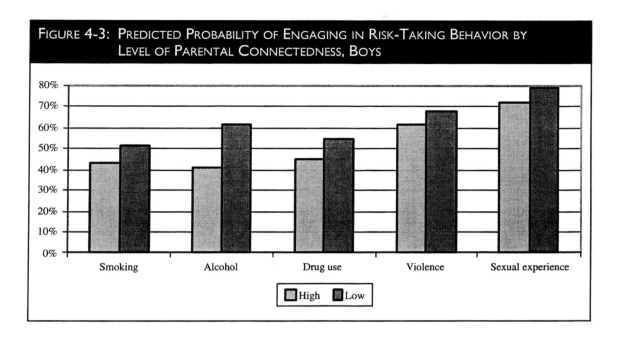

FIGURE 4-3: PREDICTED PROBABILITY OF ENGAGING IN RISK-TAKING BEHAVIOR BY LEVEL OF PARENTAL CONNECTEDNESS, BOYS

are risk factors. These can damage self-esteem; truncate a young person's personal, academic, and social development; and teach youth to perpetuate these same behaviors.

Parental connectedness: School-going youth who feel close to their parents have lower participation in substance use, violence, and sexual activity (Blum 2002). Both girls and boys who feel close to their families are about 10 percent less likely to engage in these risk-taking behaviors (figures 4-3 and 4-4). Regression results show that this is the most consistently important protective factor of those in the analysis, being positively correlated with all risk-taking behaviors (Blum 2002).

Parental connectedness is likely to directly and indirectly influence young people's decision to engage in negative behaviors. The direct influence may be a desire of the child to not disappoint caring parents. For example, young people who perceive that their parents have expectations that

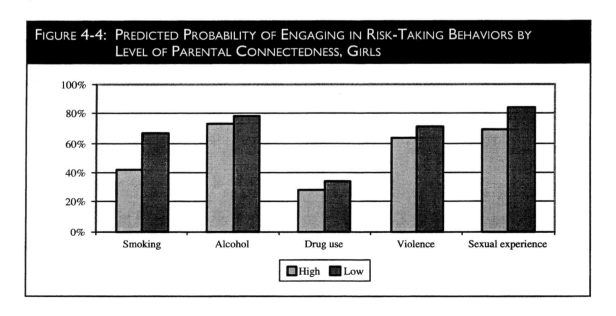

FIGURE 4-4: PREDICTED PROBABILITY OF ENGAGING IN RISK-TAKING BEHAVIORS BY LEVEL OF PARENTAL CONNECTEDNESS, GIRLS

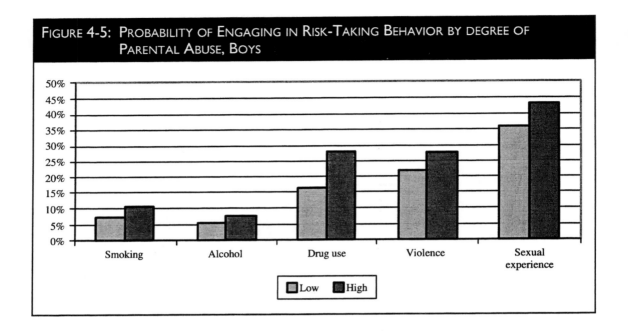

FIGURE 4-5: PROBABILITY OF ENGAGING IN RISK-TAKING BEHAVIOR BY DEGREE OF PARENTAL ABUSE, BOYS

they can complete school not only do better in school but also participate less than others in risky behaviors (Resnick and Hojat 1997, Luther, St. Ville, and Hasbún 2002). Furthermore, young people who believe that their parents would be opposed to the early onset of intercourse are less likely than their peers to become sexually active.[26] Conversely, a lack of parental connectedness leads to more rage and lower self-esteem, which drive young people toward risky behaviors.

The building blocks of parental connectedness include adult parents and resources. Interviews with youth consistently report that adolescent mothers have limited skills in being a good parent (Barker 1995, Luther, St. Ville, and Hasbún 2002) because of their inexperience in adulthood. Adolescent fathers face the same limitations as the women, but in addition, young childfathers (the father of the child of the adolescent mother) are less present and supportive than are older fathers (Russell-Brown, Engle, and Townsend 1994). Poverty also lowers parental connectedness because parents may need to spend the time working or compensating for absent public services (poor public transportation, absence of running water, absence of electricity), which precludes spending time with one's child and building a relationship.

Physical, sexual, and emotional abuse in the home: A primary risk factor that is correlated with risk-taking youth behavior is physical, sexual, and emotional abuse by parents or by nonfamily members who have access to the household. Parental abuse is correlated with higher use of alcohol and tobacco by both boys and girls, and it is even more strongly correlated with drug use, violence, and early sexual initiation. For example, 16 percent of school-going boys who are not abused by their parents use drugs, but 28 percent who are abused use drugs; for girls, drug use increases from 13 percent to 18 percent with parental abuse (figures 4-5 and 4-6). Among school-going girls, sexual experience doubles if they are abused in the home.

Child abuse can be attributed to poor parental skills, poverty, and culture. Poor parenting skills are especially relevant among adolescent parents, who have not developed as adults themselves and are unable to cope with their own children. Violence is a common response to stress and anger in Caribbean countries, feelings that may be accentuated by poverty. Moreover, scholars suggest that

---

26. Recent research suggests that most of these perceptions come from nonverbal rather than direct verbal messages (McNeely et al. forthcoming). Parental behaviors and interactions, rather than words appear to be more effective.

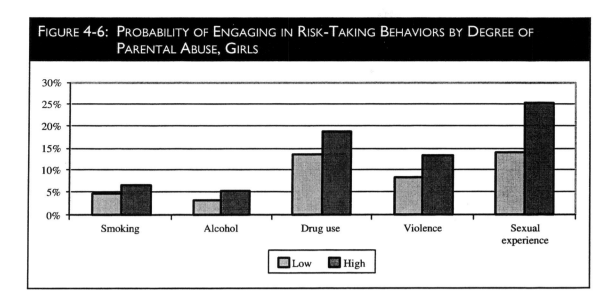

FIGURE 4-6: PROBABILITY OF ENGAGING IN RISK-TAKING BEHAVIORS BY DEGREE OF PARENTAL ABUSE, GIRLS

the acceptance of violence is reinforced through culture. Caribbean researchers hypothesize that the colonial history in the English-speaking Caribbean has institutionalized the culture of physical and mental abuse (Patterson 1975, Barrow 2001). They report that slave mothers were traditionally abusive of their children to better prepare them for their future life as slaves; sociologists suggest that this behavior is the basis of the abuse that persists today. These authors also hypothesize that men were not family fathers, serving only as biological fathers, during the slave period, so they did not feel connectedness to their own children or partners. This, in turn, lowers inhibitions against abuse by the father, making the behavior more common.

Risk-taking behavior by parents: Parental involvement in substance abuse and violence has negative demonstration effects on youth. One of the primary correlates of youth substance abuse and sexual initiation, particularly among children aged 10 to 12, is parental substance abuse(Blum 2002). The early sexual initiation may result from abusive behavior of intoxicated parents or parental friends (Barker 1995). Both violence against others and self-inflicted violence (suicide) are correlates in youth violence and suicide, especially among young children (Blum 2002).

The likely sources of risk-taking behavior by parents are from their own experiences as youth and from poverty. The intergenerational transfer of risk-taking behaviors is well known as one group of youth becomes tomorrow's problem adults and teachers of tomorrow's youth. Poverty exacerbates the situation by increasing anger and hopelessness within adults as well.

Presence of two biological parents[27]: Two-parent families have more economic and emotional resources, as well as time and energy, to devote to their children than do single parents. Single parents must both work and provide for their children's basic needs, leaving little time for deeper time and emotional investments in their children.[28] However, the presence of two adults will allow a

27. Access to extended family has also been found to be highly protective (Burton, Allison, and Obeidallah 1995). In many African tribes, it is clear to whom (other than mother or father) a young man or woman will turn in trouble. In many clans around the world, aunts and uncles are often referred to as mother and father. In highly mobile Western and migratory societies of the developing world, where young men and women leave their villages for large urban centers, this source of protection is becoming less available.

28. The youth in the focus groups and in more general consultations reflected that their mothers were their "closest friends" or had made great sacrifices for their children. Thus, this report should *not* reflect that women without partners are not good parents, nor should it suggest that their achievements are underrecognized. The report only intends to point out that the challenges are greater for a single parent and that children of single parents, even when levels of poverty are controlled for—have more difficulties than do children from two-parent households.

division of labor, resulting in higher overall family income and more time directed toward child-care.[29] This increases connectedness and thus decreases engagement in risky behaviors. According to Samms-Vaughan (2001), children have higher academic and cognitive scores when both biological parents are present, followed by two surrogate parents, and one biological parent; having a biological parent combined with a surrogate parent is associated with children's poorer academic and cognitive scores, especially when the surrogate parent is the father.[30] Samms-Vaughan hypothesizes that children's higher achievement with both biological and surrogate parents may be a result of the stability of these unions, which is transferred into the child's emotional stability.

Finally, "barrel children," whose parents have both migrated, are at a particular risk because they do not have the protection of either parent. Migration of parents is common because of better economic opportunities in other countries. Children are left behind with relatives or friends who receive payment from the parents until the parents are able to pay for passage for the children to join them. However, payment is not guaranteed and the waiting period may be very long, thus exposing young people to the influences of nonparental adults. The abandonment may lead to rage toward one's own parents, and the foster family's treatment of guest children may be particularly abusive.

Household poverty: Although higher household income does not guarantee that youth will not engage in risky behaviors, it does alleviate some of the factors that lead to the behaviors or allow families to compensate for poor choices made by the adolescent. As discussed above, poverty may lead to absent parents (either working long hours or migrants), thus breaking family connectedness. The desire to help bring resources into the household leads some youth to engage in the drug trade and the drug use and violence associated with it. In the Dominican Republic, the primary reason that poor youth cite for school dropout is to work to support the family (Luther, St. Ville, and Hasbún 2002). Even if they do not work in the drug business, youth from poor families live in neighborhoods that are drug sale points (Luther, St. Ville, and Hasbún 2002), thus surrounding youth with the negative influences. Finally, if a young person does become addicted to drugs or pregnant, poor families have few resources, especially because public services are scarce. Thus, poor youth are permanently scarred, and those from wealthier families have the resources to compensate for the negative events.

Peers, Role Models, and Social Networks

Peers, role models, and social networks can be supports to or substitutes for absent family supports. Youth choose to spend the majority of their free time with their friends. Most of these relationships are positive, but youth also identify friends and role models or protectors who lead them into risky behaviors.

Peers and social networks: Because poor (urban) youth live in violent communities where parents are often not present, gang membership was identified as a support structure, in terms of personal safety, identity, and companionship (Luther, St. Ville, and Hasbún 2002; Barker 1995). In violent neighborhoods in the Dominican Republic, for example, young people say that they are largely confined to their homes out of fear of walking in the street—simply associating with a gang provides some level of protection. Gang activities, such as drug use and sale, also give a sense of identity as a "bad boy," as they say in the Trinidad and Tobago (Barker 1995). Out-of-school boys identified peer pressure as the primary reason for their involvement in drug sales. Finally, as stated by a young man in Jamaica, "the boy does not have anyone to talk to . . . so, these youth may be bad, but at least they talk to him." (Barker 1995).

Social exclusion drives one to turn inward to one's neighborhood and social networks. As a Jamaican youth explained, "You get labeled 'inner city' . . . 'ghetto' . . . a lot of people think that ghetto is only crime and violence" (Barker 1995). This prejudice toward those who live in the poorer neighborhoods is clear in the labor market, where being from the wrong neighborhood precludes one from obtaining a job; leading to even more dependence on one's own community

---

29. Two-parent families are associated with less poverty than single-parent, mother-headed households—usually one-half to two-thirds less (Patterson and Blum 1996, Blum et al. 2000).

30. All findings were highly significant (*P*<.001) even when social class was controlled for.

(Luther, St. Ville, and Hasbún 2002). However, the community is not a stable source of support as migration continuously changes the structure of the local networks (Barker 1995).

Role models: Role models may be a protective factor, but negative role models are a risk factor. Most youth identified parents, entertainers, or teachers as role models, but drug dons are also admired for their wealth (Luther, St. Ville, and Hasbún 2002). The drug don, and his approachability and interest in recruiting children, is a particularly dangerous role model because youth easily become engaged in his business, with clear negative implications for youth behavior. Political figures were not identified as role models, instead they were identified as being "corrupt," "only for themselves," or "unworthy of their positions" (Luther, St. Ville, and Hasbún 2002).

Community and Neighborhood

The physical environment in which youth live and the institutions that they confront daily are very powerful influences on their lives. The most relevant community institutions identified are schools, the church, community organizations, and the physical neighborhood.

Schools: Similar to the finding about parental connectedness, feeling connected to school is a very powerful protective factor. Boys and girls who feel connectedness to school—through a teacher or by working hard—are 25 to 80 percent less likely to engage in risk-taking behavior than are those who do not have any connectedness. Among boys and girls without school connectedness, their participation in risky activities is as follows: 55 percent and 30 percent (respectively) use drugs, 60 and 80 percent (respectively) use alcohol, 70 percent of boys and girls are engaged in violent activity, and 80 percent of boys and girls are sexually active. Among girls and boys who feel connected to school, the probability of sexual activity falls by 30 percent for boys and 60 percent for girls (figures 4-7 and 4-8). The good school performance may not solely be due to the education system, but it is likely to also capture positive home and community support; youth say that their school attendance and performance is highly contingent on their parents' interest in their success and in monitoring their school attendance (Luther, St. Ville, and Hasbún 2002). To give credit to the school system, though, 88 percent of students feel connected to a teacher who also gives positive reinforcement. Finally, students who perform well may feel good about themselves and their future and may not want to jeopardize either by undertaking risks that may have long-term effects.

Religious organizations: Religion was identified by many youth as an important protective factor in their lives. Several interviewees in a juvenile detention center in St. Lucia identified God as

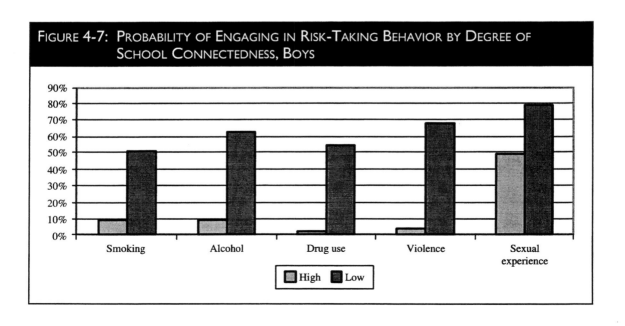

FIGURE 4-7: PROBABILITY OF ENGAGING IN RISK-TAKING BEHAVIOR BY DEGREE OF SCHOOL CONNECTEDNESS, BOYS

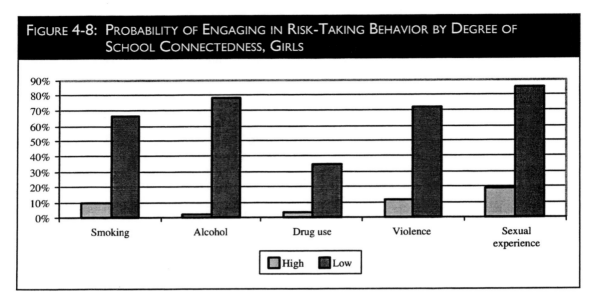

FIGURE 4-8: PROBABILITY OF ENGAGING IN RISK-TAKING BEHAVIOR BY DEGREE OF SCHOOL CONNECTEDNESS, GIRLS

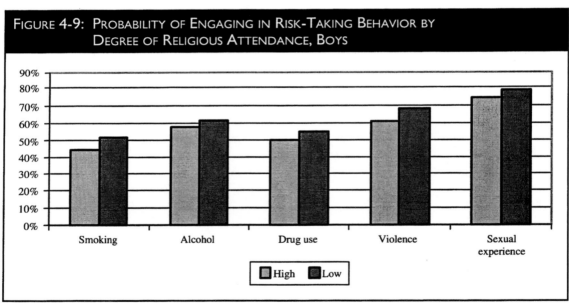

FIGURE 4-9: PROBABILITY OF ENGAGING IN RISK-TAKING BEHAVIOR BY DEGREE OF RELIGIOUS ATTENDANCE, BOYS

their primary role model, and church attendance is identified as an important activity (Luther, St. Ville, and Hasbún 2002). Thus, both individual spirituality and the act of belonging to a church community are important influences. This is supported statistically by the strong negative correlation between religious beliefs and church attendance on the one hand and substance use, violence, and sexual initiation on the other.[31] Although the magnitude of the prevention is not large, averaging a decrease of male risky behavior by 5 to 10 percent, the role of religion as a protective factor against youth negative behaviors may play a small role (figures 4-9 and 4-10). This

---

31. The odds ratios for the correlation between religious beliefs and behaviors are 0.92 for violence, 0.90 for sexual initiation, and 0.86 for substance abuse. These are particularly significant (at the 1 percent level) for those aged 13 to 15.

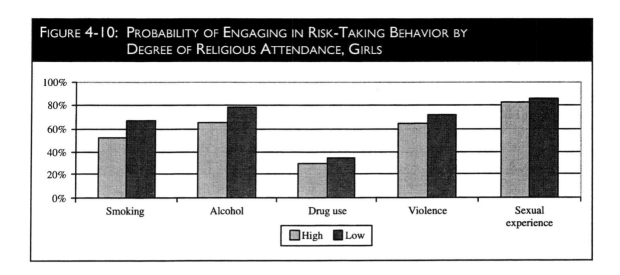

FIGURE 4-10: PROBABILITY OF ENGAGING IN RISK-TAKING BEHAVIOR BY DEGREE OF RELIGIOUS ATTENDANCE, GIRLS

may occur directly, because membership in an association is likely to be contingent on not engaging in these behaviors, or perhaps through the decreased feelings of rage in religious people.[32]

Community organizations: Youth groups and community groups are also important in the Caribbean, forming the basis of youth organization in some countries, such as the National Youth Council of St. Lucia. Although these groups play important roles in community cohesion (such as the sports club in Barbados), education (the community youth groups in Saint Lucia), or advocacy, they also have the potential to be exclusionary (Luther, St. Ville, and Hasbún 2002). For example, in the Dominican Republic, some club memberships are based on personal characteristics, such as virginity, which necessarily excludes those already at risk.

Physical environment: The neighborhood environment in which young people live can predispose them to risky behavior. For all the reasons previously expressed by the interviewees, they perceive that the environment that surrounds young people in poor communities is violent, and survival is determined by the rules of the strongest, who are usually involved in criminal activities: "Groups go about like Rambo with a knife in their mouth, trying to survive." Youth values are then distorted, and survival becomes their strongest mandate. They state that the distribution and use of drugs are common activities. Poor neighborhoods are drug distribution points that are dangerous but conducive to fast money. Gangs in these areas reign free and unhampered, always imposing rules by force. Everyone fears their actions and aggressions, and negotiations like these usually take place: "We won't tell, but don't hurt us" (Luther, St. Ville, and Hasbún 2002).

Macroenvironment

Finally, the larger environment that surrounds youth has strong influences over them that interact with the risk and protective factors at the individual and microenvironment levels. The categories of most importance for the Caribbean region, as identified by the research, are the economy; poverty and inequality; legislation and institutions; law enforcement and the judicial system; culture and history; and gender.

Economy

The nature of the small economies in many Caribbean countries is a source of risk for youth. Smaller countries cannot diversify production, so jobs are concentrated in a few industries, namely agriculture, tourism (both of which are very susceptible to international market forces), and

---

32. The odds ratio estimate of the correlation between religious beliefs and rage is 0.91 and significant at the 1 percent level.

Box 4-1: Boys in the Drug Trade—their Stories

"I had a good home . . . it's hard to get work, you need a lot of subjects in school . . . the only thing you can do is sell . . . you know, for whatever fast money." (youth, Trinidad)

"When there is . . . loss of a job (by someone at home), you see some friend out there and he has a new pair of sneakers and so you think about the easy way out. So you sell (drugs) to satisfy your ego" (youth, Trinidad)

"The standard of living may be low at home . . . and marijuana (cultivating) is a quick way of getting money" (youth, St. Vincent)

Source: Barker (1995)

---

services. This presents two challenges for youth. First, limited demand for highly skilled workers means that labor market specialization is rare and wages do not rise (Barker 1995).[33] Second, unemployment is high and job creation is low, so youth have a more difficult labor force entry experience than do youth in countries where a greater quantity and diversity of jobs exist. Even the larger, more diversified economies—like Jamaica, Trinidad and Tobago, and the Dominican Republic—have difficulties producing jobs with a living wage, leading to high youth unemployment there as well. A clear alternative is employment in the low-skilled informal sector, which is undertaken by many youth, but the market cannot absorb all labor, wages and future prospects are limited, and there is little access to financing to start one's own business, particularly for young people who have few assets to offer as collateral.[34]

As a result of these structural problems in finding jobs, the culture of migration continues. With jobs scarce and limited opportunities for higher education, the skilled labor force leaves to search for education or job opportunities elsewhere. When a young migrant with a master's degree in economics was asked why he chose to live in the United States rather than St. Lucia, his response was, "What would I do there?" Youth are giving up on their countries, searching elsewhere for the support and the lifestyles they cannot get at home.

Some youth who do not migrate find the combination of youth unemployment and poverty pushing them to work in the drug trade, which has a high demand for unskilled labor. The Caribbean region is increasingly used as a drug transshipment port between Latin America and the United States or Europe (UNDCP 1997). The scarcity and low pay of legal jobs, the attraction of the "easy money," laws protecting those under age 18 from prison (Luther, St. Ville, and Hasbún 2002), and the marketing to youth by drug dons (Barker 1995) make this job opportunity very attractive to youth.

Poverty and Inequality

Youth from poor areas identify poverty as a key source of risky behaviors. Interviews reveal that young men and women feel that they need to work to support their families (Luther, St. Ville, and Hasbún 2002). Given their low levels of education, especially if they have been excluded from the education system by earning low examination marks, they have few options except informal sector work, the drug trade, or commercial sex work or sexual exploitation (Barker 1995).[35] Also, the lack of income leads to parental absence and aggression, which has implications for youth behaviors.

---

33. Jobs do exist, but youth do not feel that they are fairly remunerated. For example, a young unemployed man in Jamaica explained, "There are lots of places that want to pay you nothing [for working]. They use and abuse you" (Barker 1995).

34. The difficulty of access to financing to start small firms is recognized by many organizations in the region. Efforts are being made by international organizations (such as the Commonwealth Youth Programme, Caribbean Region) and local NGOs (such as the Barbados Youth Business Trust) to provide low-interest loans and support services to young entrepreneurs.

35. Increasingly, the public health field refers to prostitution of adults as sex work or commercial sex work and prostitution of children and adolescents younger than age 18 as sex exploitation.

Interviews with young, uneducated, poor women in Jamaica reveal that they fully understand reproductive health, but their best income prospects are from pregnancy and child support (Barker 1995). Finally, the income inequality demonstrated by drug dons, foreign tourists, and the media encourages the engagement in the "easy money" activities, including drugs and prostitution (Barker 1995; Luther, St. Ville, and Hasbún 2002).

Public Policy and Institutions

The education system: The existing education system in the English-speaking Caribbean countries was inherited from the British colonial education system in both structure and content. Students are exposed to technical and vocational subjects only when they are deemed as unable to perform academically, effectively categorizing technical-vocational students as an underclass.

The structure of the educational system directly induces risky behavior. The Common Entrance Examinations (CEEs) in most English-speaking countries of the Caribbean are a clear threat to young people because their performance on these exams determines their worth to society. Those who pass the exam—a term that is not entirely correct because the passing score is a function of the number of places available in secondary school, not necessarily a minimum level of competency—are implicitly told that they are valuable to society and are permitted entrance to the next level, which improves their probability of success later in life, thus having a positive effect on self-esteem and discouraging risk-taking behaviors.[36] However, those who enter secondary school are not free from judgment because school placement is based on the points achieved from the CEEs. Consequently, youth define themselves and each other based on the uniform they wear and the school they attend.[37] The sense of achievement of having made it through this competitive process adds to their self-worth, and conversely it hurts those who do not pass. Students from the focus groups with the highest sense of self-worth and confidence were those who had achieved tertiary-level education. Thus, the system *induces* risk-taking behavior by forcing children to leave. Those who do not pass the exams are effectively told that they do not have value and that the government's investment in them, and in their futures, ends at a young age. This rejection and denial of opportunities that will lead to a successful life understandably lead to rage, depression, and negative behaviors. This is particularly acute among youth from poor families, who have fewer resources and opportunities for adequate preparation to perform well on the CEEs.

In both the Dominican Republic and the English-speaking Caribbean, youth felt that the school curriculum was not appropriate to prepare them for the labor market. A Youth Senator in Saint Lucia describes the curriculum as having an academic bias that develops no talent or skill in students and does not nurture them so that they can make a meaningful contribution to the society. He described the quality and the dimensions of education now on offer as unsuited for the economic and social realities of our time. Students are taught academics to prepare them for the future without them having tangible employment prospects, and with them also lacking any marketable skills or any entrepreneurial spirit. Further, academically strong youth are confronted by the inability of their impressive academic certificates to ease their entry into a good job. Activities like drug dealing and other profitable criminal activities, as well as migration, become viable options to meet their expectations of personal success.

Classrooms are sources of violent conflict. At-risk youth, especially males, voiced negative views of teachers and authority figures within the education system. Even though most youth (88 percent [Blum 2002]) feel connected to a teacher, youth report the unfairness of corporal punishment and physical fights with teachers (Williams 2001). Males, in particular, felt that they were being ostracized and were not provided with adequate support by teachers. Of greatest con-

---

36. The system is perhaps more egalitarian but also damaging in the rural Dominican Republic, where there are not enough spaces for all secondary school–age students. This is solved by some students leaving school on their own choice (Luther, St. Ville, and Hasbun 2002).

37. All St. Lucian secondary students wear different school uniforms that allow societal differentiation of students and further aids the development of academic elitism and discrimination.

cern was the teachers' ability to arbitrarily punish and report to parents. Another issue that further alienates at-risk youth is the holding back of low-achievers. The students are held up to ridicule by their peers, leaving youth prone to truancy and eventual dropout from the educational system (Luther, St. Ville, and Hasbún 2002).

Immigrant children are systematically excluded from the school system. In the Dominican Republic and St. Martin, for example, the requirement of national birth certificates for school enrollment and under provision of schools in immigrant neighborhoods completely exclude these most vulnerable children and youth from the system. When this is combined with unstructured free time, poverty, and absent parents, these youth are particularly vulnerable to risky behaviors (Barker 1995, World Bank 2001a).

The health care system: Youth interviewed cite lack of confidentiality as a key risk factor in seeking health care services. Problems related to the health care facilities are particularly important, given high levels of HIV/AIDS, low contraceptive use among sexually active adolescents, and teenage pregnancy. According to a review of international experiences in the provision of services to at-risk youth, health care programs tended to lack youth-sensitive services (Barker and Fontes 1996). Given that many of the health problems youth face are sensitive (e.g., sexuality), having primary and secondary health care professionals who understand the needs of youth is critical to reducing risky behavior related to adolescent health.

Law Enforcement and the Judiciary

Youth in the Dominican Republic and St. Lucia are untrusting of the legal and judicial systems in their neighborhoods. They report that police are prejudiced against youth and treat them badly. This is particularly the case in poor neighborhoods, where police assume that all youth are engaged in the drug trade or crime. Youth feel that police fail at their jobs of providing security—instead, drug dons run the neighborhoods, especially after dark. A similar distrust is felt of the judicial and more general political system, where youth feel that all authorities are corrupt and untrustworthy.

Culture and History

Aggression, substance use, and adolescent childbirth in the contemporary Caribbean region are the legacy of colonialism and the system of slave labor that fuelled its sugarcane-based plantation economy. Attitudes toward alcohol, violence, and family continue to be informed by social norms formed during the colonial era. For example, now as then, alcohol is not seen as a drug (Luther, St. Ville, and Hasbún 2002), and many consider its consumption an integral cultural activity. As one Barbadian said, "We grow sugarcane here; everyone drinks rum—they always have." Marijuana is similarly seen as a social drug that is medicinal and not harmful or immoral (Barker 1995).[38]

Physical violence, whether in the homes or schools, may also be attributed to the colonial experience, especially in the English-speaking Caribbean countries. As discussed above, the school system is based on the English system, in which corporal punishment is an element of school discipline. This system survived colonialism and institutionalized certain forms of violence that are often not questioned today. Violence in the home by the mother is also identified as a form of discipline. Some historical anthropologists attribute it to the slave mother disciplining her children in the manner in which they would be disciplined when they began working. Finally, domestic violence by men is accepted as a gender role.

The structure of the household in the English-speaking Caribbean is also traced back to conditions of slavery. Families were discouraged because they would be broken up in the sale of slaves, but women were encouraged to bear many children (capital production for the slave owner). Thus,

---

38. Despite the cultural acceptance of marijuana, it is illegal in the Caribbean region. In the 13-country data collection exercise by PAHO, marijuana use was reported by fewer than 2 percent of school-going children—a very unlikely statistic. The researcher opined that the respondents may have underreported use because of the illegality of the narcotic.

men were excluded from the family and were not encouraged to be participating fathers. The high number of out-of-wedlock births, the propensity for men to float among several partners, and the absence of expectations for men to be responsible partners and fathers persists today and leads to unstable family situations. The many challenges faced by women without a partner often set up conditions for children to engage in risky behaviors.

The household in the Dominican Republic is very different, with a single, tight family in which family honor is paramount. This does not imply that single-mother households do not exist, but the incidence of men who float among many households is less prevalent. However, single mother-hood is more of a stigma in this highly Catholic country, where pregnant, unmarried daughters are regularly expelled from the household or treated as domestic servants in return for living with their children in their parents' house. This familial exclusion leads to risky conditions for young mothers (Luther, St. Ville, and Hasbún 2002).

Gender

Gender is a risk factor for Caribbean male and female adolescents, as evidenced by the differenti-ated outcomes realized by boys and girls. For example, male school-going students were much more likely to report violence involvement than females (odds ratios for 10- to 12-year-olds: 2.37; for 13- to 15-year-olds: 2.96; and for 16- to 18-year-olds: 3.03). Boys were also twice as likely as girls to report having had sexual intercourse, less likely than girls to report suicide attempts, and consistently more likely to report rage for every age group of teens (Blum 2002).

Gender norms and values may lead to negative outcomes. Men's masculinities are often mea-sured by their abilities to provide economically for their partners and children, a challenge made more difficult in recent years by continued high unemployment in many countries, feminization of certain sectors (e.g., manufacturing), and a general cynicism about prospects for future work (Lewis forthcoming). Although these changes have sometimes worked to dislocate dominant gender roles—providing some avenues for increased participation by women in the public realm, for example—they have often resulted in the ostracizing of some fathers by their children for fail-ing to meet their responsibilities and pushed other men to look to illicit activities (violence and drug dealing) as a means of earning an income. As fathers hold enormous influence over their children's choices—as one study on the effects of early childbearing in Barbados showed, fathers' close relationship with children was associated with higher academic achievement (Russell-Brown, Engle, and Townsend 1994)—and both fathers' absence and their involvement in high-risk activities can fundamentally shape young peoples' lives.

Caribbean men's masculinities are also often tied to display of physical bravado, engagement in violence (Barker 1998), and sexual prowess (Barriteau 2001), thus providing an unhealthy tem-plate of high-risk behavior for younger adolescents. For example, some Jamaican men have rejected condom use on the grounds that "real men" prefer to "ride bare back" (World Bank 2001b).

Gender norms are also a risk factor for women. For example, higher rates of sexual abuse of girls represent a fundamental risk factor for females. Moreover, men's inability to meet the expecta-tion of being an economic provider means that a large proportion of women raise children on their own, leading to greater levels of poverty and vulnerability among these women and their children. The children of single mothers are also more likely to go unsupervised and be exposed to negative peer groups that prey on children (e.g., gang leaders). The expectation that women will be more passive than men means that women have a more difficult time negotiating condom use, thereby exposing them to HIV/AIDs and other STIs.

Interconnectedness of Factors

Risk-taking behaviors are highly correlated, meaning that individuals who engage in one type of risk-taking behavior are likely to engage in several risk-taking behaviors. Although this analysis did not explicitly test for a bundling of risk-taking behaviors, the repeated influence of the same factors and the high participation in risk-taking behaviors of youth without any protective factors (or with

TABLE 4-2: PREDICTED PROBABILITIES THAT A CARIBBEAN YOUTH WILL BE VIOLENT BASED ON DEGREE OF PROTECTIVE FACTORS, BY GENDER					
Number of protective factors	Family connectedness	Religious attendance	School connectedness	Males (%)	Females (%)
0	Low	Low	Low	68.1	71.9
1	High	Low	Low	61.9	63.9
	Low	High	Low	60.7	64.1
	Low	Low	High	39.9	11.6
2	High	High	Low	54.0	55.2
	Low	High	High	32.4	8.4
	High	Low	High	33.6	8.3
3	High	High	High	26.7	5.9

multiple risk factors) suggests that bundling of risk-taking behaviors occurs in the Caribbean region. Thus, public policy that focuses on reducing a single risk factor will have wide-reaching implications for several different types of behaviors, and focused preventive measures may be an efficient means to simultaneously address several different types of risk-taking behavior.

However, it is unclear which preventive measure to invest in because the marginal impact of each factor cannot be disentangled. Multiple protective factors decrease the propensity for a young person to engage in risk-taking behavior, but it is difficult to identify the exact impact of each factor.[39] For example (table 4-2), 72 percent of girls with low family, religious, and school connectedness are violent. Violence among girls falls to 64 percent if family connectedness is high, to 64 percent if religious attendance is high, and 12 percent if only school connectedness is high. However, among girls with all three types of connectedness, only 6 percent are violent. The result that the total effect is not the sum of the individual effects suggests that there are correlated underlying influences among the three types of connectedness. From a policy perspective, focusing on enhancing a single protective factor will have great impacts. It may not be necessary to address all protective and risk factors initially, but instead to identify those bundles that are most successful at lowering the risk.

Final Thoughts

Youth respond to the incentives and environments that are taught and presented to them, suggesting that youth themselves are not the problem. Instead, the environment in which they exist and their support structures either force risky conditions upon them, such as school leaving for young, English-speaking Caribbean students who do not do well on their CEEs, or set up conditions where engagement in risky behavior is a reasonable option, such as the case of the drug trade when unemployment is rampant. There is also a high degree of interconnectedness among the different risk or protective categories, suggesting the potential value of a more holistic approach to working with youth to improve their situations. However, parental involvement, both emotional and a physical presence, is one of the most important protective factors. Unfortunately, as a result of the changing economy, migration, and socialization, this resource is even scarcer.

---

39. Ideally, this would be accomplished in a multivariate regression, but high collinearity among the factors precludes this option.

5

THE COSTS OF RISKY ADOLESCENT BEHAVIOR

The negative outcomes of risky youth behaviors impose costs not only on young people and their families, but also on the economy and society at large. This chapter estimates the cost to individuals and society of school dropouts, risky sexual behavior resulting in adolescent pregnancy, risky sexual behavior resulting in youth HIV/AIDS, youth unemployment, and youth crime and violence in as many countries as the data permit.[40] The numbers presented in this chapter are, at best, rough and conservative estimates of the costs of risky adolescent behavior to society because full measurement would require impossible tasks of putting a price on life, quantifying the psychological and social costs of risky behavior, and identifying and measuring all the externalities of the behaviors in both observed and future periods.[41] Furthermore, missing or unavailable data result in underestimates of those costs that should be measurable. Thus, the costs presented are only a *lower bound;* the total costs of the behaviors are much higher. Despite these underestimates, it is clear that costs to individuals and society reach into the billions of dollars.

Social and private economic and financial costs for each behavior are estimated and/or discussed:

■ *Financial costs* are those line items in government or private budgets. However, these may not be a cost to society as a whole because they are a transfer from one individual to another, with no net loss of resources to society.

■ *Economic costs* are those costs that create a net loss to society through the forgone value of the productive input, also known as the *opportunity cost* of the resource. In other words, economic

---

40. Cross-country comparisons should not be made because the sources of the data used for each country differ, thus not making them comparable.

41. Placing a monetary cost on the outcomes of human behavior may be distasteful because it collapses complex human behaviors into prices and uses labor productivity to put a value on a person's life. Ideally, some measure of happiness would be used, but such a metric does not commonly exist, so currency values, though imperfect, are used instead.

costs are measured as the benefits not realized either as a result of direct actions, such as lost family income because the primary breadwinner is in prison, or as a result of an alternative use of resources, such as better child nutrition that is not realized because resources are spent on drug treatment programs for adolescents rather than for school lunches.[42]

The methodology for this chapter is to measure the productive value of the human and monetary resources and the measurable costs associated with various behaviors. The chapter differentiates between *social costs*—those that are borne by society as a whole—and *private costs* that are borne only by the young person him- or herself. The methodology for the cost estimates is given in appendix 2.

This chapter does not generate cost-benefit estimates. To carry out a cost-benefit analysis, specific program costs and outcomes from the program are needed. This chapter does not consider the program costs, but instead calculates only the resources that are lost to negative outcomes from risk-taking behaviors by youth.

The chapter also does not estimate all the individual and social costs of youth behaviors, nor does it generate estimates for all countries considered. Only a subset of behaviors is analyzed; these behaviors were selected based on data availability. This is not to suggest that drug use, early marriage by women, child labor, poor nutritional status, sexual activity that results in STIs, and physical or sexual abuse of youth, among others, are not important costs, only that they are more difficult to measure. Additionally, the choice of countries was solely based on data availability and is not a judgment of the prevalence of the costly outcomes or the extent and manner in which the countries are addressing the issue.

Crime and Violence

The total cost of crime committed by youth cannot be accurately estimated because many of the crimes include immeasurable losses, such as those resulting from murder, sexual offenses, and drug trafficking. Furthermore, criminal activity at a young age has long-term implications for a person's future criminal activity and his or her integration into society. However, some rough tools can be used to conservatively estimate the social and private costs of crime and violence.

At a minimum, the following would be needed to conservatively calculate the financial and economic costs of juvenile crime and violence:

- *Arrest, prosecution, and detention of criminals:* The total expenditure on these activities would enumerate the financial costs to society. Economic costs will differ, being measured as the forgone benefits from spending these resources on arrest, prosecution, and detention of criminals rather than on alternative government investments.
- *Property loss and damage:* This is a clear financial cost. The economic costs differ, though, because robbery may be considered a transfer of goods from one individual to another, thus not having social costs. However, property damage or the psychological costs of being robbed do impose real costs on society (Roman and Farrell 2001).
- *Medical costs, public programs for victims, and lost income of the victim:* resources to aid the victims of crimes are both a financial and an economic cost to society, the individual victim, or the family of the criminal. Measurement of these costs is difficult, particularly the value

---

42. For example, economic costs include the forgone labor market output of youth who are in prison, and financial estimates would not include this as a cost. Alternatively, government transfers to teenaged mothers would be a financial cost (which would show up on government accounts), but they are not economic costs because society *as a whole* does not gain or lose—the benefits simply move from one person to another (assuming that the joy in the goods purchased by the teenaged mother with this money is equal to the unhappiness of the person whose taxes paid for the transfer). Instead, the economic cost of the transfer is the lost effects of the alternative use of the transfer—for example, an additional healthy day for a person with HIV if the transfer were used instead to treat an opportunistic infection.

of a lost life, but average victim compensation values, based on jury awards in the United States, allow a conservative estimate (Roman and Farrell 2001), as given in table 5-1.

▓ *Intangible costs (pain, suffering, and quality of life):* Courts recognize the nonpecuniary costs of a crime by awarding damages to compensate for pain and suffering. Although these private costs are difficult to quantify, estimates derived from victim compensation court awards place a conservative value on the psychological damages caused by crime. The large magnitude of these estimates demonstrates the large private cost to the victim or to the victim's family (in the case of murder), which may be interpreted as the net cost to social well-being.

▓ *Security costs:* Expenditures on deterrence mechanisms clearly divert resources from other productive uses. The government and private expenditures on security are clearly identifiable. However, forgone benefits are also real costs of investment in personal and public security. Financial support of a police force, monitoring cameras, urban street lights, and other security measures divert resources from other productive uses. Similarly, private expenditures on security guards, fences to surround property, and security systems do not return rewards from alternative uses of the resources.

▓ *Lower tourist receipts:* Unquestionably, the Caribbean region benefits from tourism, but crime and violence decrease the demand for this service by potential tourists (Levantis and Gani 2000). The forgone tourist earnings are quite costly for the government as tax receipts from tour ships, airports, and tourist services decrease. The economic costs at the level of the individual are also quite high because lower demand in the tourist sector leads to unemployment and a lower standard of living.

▓ *Lost income:* While a juvenile delinquent is in the legal system or prison, he or she cannot provide income to his or her family, which is likely to have made an investment in the young person. This forgone income may be costly to the individual's family (though the degree is likely to be low because unemployment is so high among young people). Additionally, the state loses the taxes from the labor income and/or consumption of the juvenile delinquent.

▓ *Lost social capital:* A person who is known as a criminal is likely to have less social capital in mainstream society but more in the less savory sectors of society. A loss of social capital suggests a difficult time finding work, obtaining credit (formal or informal), starting a legitimate business, being a neighbor, participating in community activities, and contributing to general society. However, social capital with those engaged in criminal activity is likely to increase, offering opportunities that involve more serious risk-taking behaviors.

Quantification of the many costs is impossible because of the difficulty of measuring some of the concepts or missing data. However, pulling together data from various countries will allow some rough, conservative estimates of the private and social economic costs of crime and violence.

TABLE 5-1: VICTIM COMPENSATION FOR TANGIBLE AND INTANGIBLE COSTS OF CRIMES, UNITED STATES

Crime	Tangible costs[a]	Intangible costs[b]
Murder	–	$1,910,000
Rape and sexual assault	$5,100	$81,400
Robbery or attempt with injury	$5,200	$13,800
Assault or attempt	$1,500	$7,800
Burglary or attempt	$1,100	$300

a. Tangible costs include medical costs, lost earnings, and public programs for victims.
b. Intangible costs include pain, suffering and quality-of-life compensation.
Source: Roman and Farrell 2001.

TABLE 5-2: ESTIMATED ECONOMIC COST OF YOUTH CRIME, IN LOCAL CURRENCY				
	Jamaica		St. Lucia	
	Social	Private	Social	Private
Total cost of youth crime	J$96 million	J$2.5 billion	EC$8.5 million	EC$208 million
Cost of youth crime as % of GDP	0.04%	0.92%	0.45%	11.01%
Marginal cost of youth crime (burglary)	J$21,000	J$61,000	EC$2,000	EC$7,000
Marginal cost of youth crime (sexual assault)	J$30,000	J$3 million	EC$2,700	EC$226,000

Source: Author's calculations; see appendix for data sources of each component.

Social financial costs: Data for Trinidad and Tobago show that the most basic social financial cost of a crime amounts to TT$31,500 (about US$5,000) per person arrested, which can be disaggregated into arrest (TT$11,196), court appearances (TT$11,104), and six months of incarceration ($TT9,205) (World Bank 1996). Additional data from the United States, which estimates the victim compensation values of medical care, public programs for victims, and lost earnings (although the last item is not a social cost, it could not be extracted from the total sums), suggest that another US$1,100 to $5,100 is spent in public funds per crime committed (table 5-1). Using youth crime data from Jamaica and St. Lucia, a conservative estimate of annual government expenditures in tangible costs amounts to approximately US$33 million for Jamaica and US$25 million for St. Lucia. Assuming that arrest, court appearances, and detention costs and durations in St. Lucia and Jamaica are similar to those in Trinidad and Tobago, the total social financial cost from youth crimes, even before including the cost of the police force, is approximately US$39 million in Jamaica and US$46 million in St. Lucia.[43]

Private financial costs: Using data from Trinidad and Tobago, rough estimates of out-of-pocket private financial costs may be estimated. Expenditures by citizens to protect themselves from being victims of the crimes is estimated to be US$3,696 per household per lifetime in fixed costs and an additional annual expenditure of US$1,200 to US$30,000. The cost of property loss or damage could not be estimated from the available data.

Social economic costs: The absence of arrest and prosecution data for Trinidad and Tobago does not permit the calculation of the annual economic costs of youth crime to Trinidadian and Tobagonian citizens and taxpayers, but prosecution data from Jamaica and Barbados allow a rough estimate. The total social economic cost of youth crime is more than J$96 million dollars in Jamaica and more than EC$8.5 million in St. Lucia (columns 1 and 3 in table 5-2), equivalent to 0.04 percent of gross domestic product (GDP) in Jamaica and 0.45 percent of GDP in St. Lucia.[44] However, it should be remembered that these are underestimates of the true social costs because the they do not include such items as forgone social capital, underinvestment in youth, impacts on the children of criminals, depletion of the juvenile delinquent's human capital, and mental health implications, for example.

---

43. The difference in estimates between these two countries is due to higher tangible costs in Jamaica but a larger number of youth prosecuted and incarcerated in St. Lucia. This is not to suggest that St. Lucia is more violent than Jamaica, but only that the prosecution rates of youth in St. Lucia exceed those of Jamaica. The prosecution **rates** for Jamaica are from Pantin (2000) and those for St. Lucia are from *Social Policy in St. Lucia* (2000).

44. The social economic cost is the sum of forgone taxes of the young person while he or she is in prison; forgone use of resources for prosecution, arrest, and detention (assuming that these are of a similar magnitude as in Trinidad and Tobago); and forgone benefits of resources used for victim assistance (assuming the magnitudes are similar to victim compensation in the United States).

TABLE 5-3: ESTIMATED INCREASE IN TOURIST FLOWS AND EXPENDITURES DUE TO A 1 PERCENT DECREASE IN YOUTH CRIME		
	Jamaica	**Bahamas**
Number of new tourists	45,920	36,340
Total new earnings due to more tourists	US$40,680,911	US$31,943,672
New earnings as % of tourism receipts	4.01	2.34

Source: Tourist flows and receipts from the Caribbean Tourism Organization; number of crimes from the U.N.; author's calculations.

An additional item that is not included in table 5-2 is the cost of crime to the tourist industry. Crime is a deterrent to tourism, one of the most important industries in many Caribbean countries. Recent research shows that a 1 percent increase in the crime rate reduced tourist flows by one-half to three-quarters percent (Levantis and Gani 2000). Applying these parameters to youth crime, if youth crime decreases by 1 percent, the tourist flows to Jamaica and the Bahamas will increase by more than 45,000 and 36,000 tourists per year, respectively. This is equivalent to more than US$40 million in Jamaica and US$31 million in the Bahamas, a 4.0 percent and 2.3 percent increase in tourist revenues, respectively (table 5-3).

Private economic costs: The private economic costs of crime far outweigh the social costs.[45] The total private economic costs to citizens of juvenile crime are EC$208 million in St. Lucia and J$2.5 billion in Jamaica *each year* (columns 2 and 4 of table 5-2). This is equivalent to 11 percent and 0.92 percent of GDP, respectively. The private costs far exceed the public costs for two primary reasons. First, victims realize the full, intangible, private economic costs, which are particularly high, and the state only realizes the benefits of an alternative use of tangible resources. For example, the J$2.9 million difference in the private costs between a burglary and a sexual offense in Jamaica, as given in table 5-2, is solely due to the different value placed on the pain and suffering by the victim of each type of crime. The marginal private cost between burglary and sexual offenses differs by EC$219,000 in St. Lucia. Second, the family of the juvenile delinquent experiences the full loss of income, and the state realizes only a portion of that in lost tax revenues. However, it should be noted that the state costs of crime are likely to be severely underestimated because of the lack of data on the cost of police protection and other preventive measures

Risk-Taking Sexual Activity: Adolescent Pregnancy[46]

The cost of adolescent pregnancy includes not only the immediate needs of the mother and child, but also the costs to their family, the father and his family, taxpayers, and society. These costs are not limited to the birth period, but include both financial costs—which are paid by the mother, family, or taxpayers over the life of the mother and child—and economic costs in the form of forgone earnings of the mother and the child when he or she becomes an adult and the loss of the benefits of alternative uses of the transfers to support adolescent mothers and their children. The additional costs incurred by a new mother who is an adolescent, rather than and adult, may include:

- *Lower lifetime earnings of the mother:* Lifetime earnings may be lower for adolescent mothers as a result of early school dropout, fewer opportunities for advanced education because of

---

45. The private costs presented in table 5-2 are the sum of the psychological (intangible) costs of crime and the forgone income from an alternative use of money spent on security (assuming that the fixed and variable costs are paid once someone has been a victim)—both of which accrue to the victim—and the forgone earnings of the juvenile delinquent, which is a cost to the family of the criminal.

46. The method for calculating costs in this section was developed by Maynard (1996).

to poverty (single mothers tend to be poorer) and childcare demands, fewer employment options because of childcare demands, and less accumulated job market experience because mothers exit the labor market often, thus slowing down their human capital accumulation. Evidence from the United States shows that teenaged mothers have *higher* lifetime earnings than women who are in their early 20ss when they bear children; this is attributed to longer work hours of young mothers because they are often the sole provider for the child (Maynard 1996). However, evidence from Barbados suggests the opposite: Adolescent mothers earn 22 percent less than do women who have children at an older age, primarily because of earlier school dropout of adolescent mothers (Russell-Brown, Engle, and Townsend 1994).[47] They are as likely to be employed. This is largely a private cost.

■ *Lower tax revenues:* The parallel social cost to lower income among adolescent mothers is the forgone tax revenue that would have been collected from a woman who delayed childbirth. The lost tax revenue may have been collected through income or consumption taxes.

■ *Fewer remarriage possibilities:* Virginity before marriage is valued in some countries, thus adolescent pregnancy may decrease the likelihood of ever marrying, which increases household poverty. An opinion survey from the Dominican Republic shows that 65 percent of youth believe that a woman should be a virgin upon marriage (Tejada, Herold and Morris 1992). However, this does not necessarily disproportionately affect union formation by adolescent mothers in all countries; in Barbados, for example, teenaged mothers were no less likely to form a union than were older women (Russell-Brown, Engle, and Townsend 1994). Again, this cost largely accrues to the mother and her child—a private cost—but society may pay a financial cost in the form of transfers to the poor households or an economic cost in forgone benefits to alternative transfer programs.

■ *Child support:* Teen mothers are less likely to receive child support from the childfathers than are mothers of older children because the adolescent fathers are more likely to be absent, which increases household poverty. Adolescent women tend to have young partners, whose earnings ability is low and who are likely to form unions elsewhere (in the Dominican Republic, nearly 30 percent of adolescent boys have more than one sex partner [Tejada 1992]). In Barbados, 44 percent of fathers of children whose mother was an adolescent when she gave birth pay child support, compared with more than 60 percent of men whose children have older mothers (Russell-Brown, Engle, and Townsend 1994). The mother, her family, and society thus share the burden of supporting the child. Because child support is a transfer, it carries clear financial costs, but the economic costs are confined to the forgone benefits of the resources that are spent in the legal system to assign and monitor child support payments. This is likely to be a small value, though, because monitoring is a rare activity in most Caribbean countries.

■ *Higher health care costs:* Complications in births to teenaged mothers are more common because young women's bodies are less developed to cope with the stress of childbirth. Also, children of adolescent mothers tend to have more health problems (Maynard 1996). This imposes financial costs not only on the mother and her family, but also on the public health system. Economic costs are again measured by the forgone benefits of the alternative use of the private and public funds that are used to administer and provide health care to adolescent mothers and their children.

■ *Disadvantaged children:* As a result of the higher poverty rate among teen mothers and the absence of a father figure, many children of teenaged parents tend to have more behavioral problems (Russell-Brown, Engle, and Townsend 1994), less educational attainment (Russell-Brown, Engle, and Townsend 1994), a higher likelihood of being teenaged parents them-

---

47. The results for Barbados should be taken as a rough estimate because the analysis did not control for the age difference between adolescent mothers and nonadolescent mothers, which will affect earnings, and characteristics that decrease earnings and are correlated with adolescent pregnancy.

TABLE 5-4: ESTIMATED SOCIAL COSTS OF ADOLESCENT PREGNANCY RELATIVE TO YOUNG ADULT PREGNANCY, US$

Type of cost	Annual per birth, US$		Annual per cohort, thousands of US$		Lifetime per cohort, millions of US$	
	Financial	Economic	Financial	Economic	Financial	Economic
Barbados	262	303	118	137	4.6	6.4
Dominican Republic	60	165	2,595	7,130	85.8	336.3
Guyana	28	33	28	34	1.0	1.6
Jamaica	122	167	587	805	22.2	38.0
St. Kitts and Nevis	234	363	33	51	1.1	2.4
St. Lucia	98	162	55	91	1.8	4.3
Trinidad and Tobago	130	216	156	260	5.0	12.6

Note: Excludes the forgone earnings of the child when he or she is an adult in the labor force; adding this cost was too subjective.

Source: Wages from the ILO, cost of social programs from the World Bank (1996), cost of incarceration from the World Bank (1996), incarceration rates from the U.N., health care costs from PAHO (1999) and teen pregnancy totals from PAHO (1999).

selves (Maynard 1996), and a higher likelihood of engaging in violent crime (Grogger as cited in Maynard 1996, World Bank 1996). These contribute to higher poverty for the child when he or she becomes an adult—a private financial and economic cost—as well as lower productivity in society, lower tax revenues, higher crime costs, and fewer contributions to society at large, which affect both government balance sheets and economic costs. Furthermore, the higher poverty rate will likely result in a transfer of these behaviors to their own children, thus repeating the cycle of high financial and economic costs.

▪ *Higher demands on the social system:* The poverty associated with teen pregnancy and the expulsion of young mothers from their family households lead to an increased demand for foster care, government transfers, children's nutritional programs, food programs, and government housing (Maynard 1996). These transfers are clear financial costs, but they also create economic costs through the forgone benefits of alternative program supports.

▪ *Social exclusion and poor mental health:* Young, unmarried women who give birth may be cast out of their household and community, such as has been noted in the Dominican Republic, which makes them less successful in integrating into productive society, creating both private and social economic costs.

To estimate the cost of adolescent childbirth, the above concepts are categorized into four groups: private financial costs, social financial costs, private economic costs, and social economic costs.[48] Only social costs are presented in table 5-4 because few measures of private costs were available. Three estimates are presented for each economic (or financial) cost by country: annual cost per birth, annual cost for all births in a year, and lifetime costs for all births in a single year. The costs are estimated for the mother's age (15 to 19 years) compared with new mothers in their early 20s, thus these costs are not the total cost to the young women of raising their chil-

---

48. Social financial costs are the sum of the additional health costs of adolescent mothers and their children, the value of government transfers, the expected financial costs of crime committed by the children, and the cost of child support. The economic social costs are given by the forgone tax revenue and the forgone benefit of alternative uses of resources spent on health care, transfers, and criminality of adolescent mothers and/or their children. A discount rate of 6 percent is used in the calculation of lifetime costs.

dren but instead are the additional costs that accrue to the mothers because they gave birth during adolescence.

The net social financial cost over the lifetime of a single cohort of adolescent mothers in the Caribbean region ranges from US$1 million in Guyana to US$86 million in the Dominican Republic. These costs are particularly large in the Dominican Republic and Jamaica because of the larger size of the population in these countries and the higher number of teen births. However, the cost per pregnancy is highest elsewhere. The social financial costs, which include health care, government transfers, financial costs of crime committed by the children, and child support, average from US$28 per year per birth to US$262 per year per birth. The high costs in Barbados and St. Kitts and Nevis are attributable to higher child support payments by the father (which are a function of wages), more generous government transfers, and the higher cost of healthcare; these costs are low in Guyana.

The net social economic cost over the lifetime of one cohort of adolescent mothers ranges from US$1.6 million in Guyana to more than US$335 million in the Dominican Republic (table 5-4). The sum of forgone tax revenues, the opportunity cost of the criminality of the children when they become adults, and the forgone benefits from spending government transfers and health care on others averages from US$33 annually in Guyana to US$363 annually in St. Kitts. Again, the large disparity is due to differences in wages and generosity of government expenditures among Caribbean countries. But as in the financial cost estimates, those countries with the largest populations have the largest total bill because of higher numbers of teen pregnancies. It should also be noted that the economic costs are much higher than the financial costs, but most of the cost of adolescent childbirth is privately born, so the social costs presented here, although large, far underestimate the cost to mothers and families.

Risk-Taking Sexual Activity: HIV/AIDS

The cost of HIV/AIDS attributable to youth is difficult to measure because the period between contraction of the illness and appearance of symptoms may be anywhere from 5 to 10 years. The majority of new HIV/AIDS cases are not reported by youth, but rather are reported by those in the age group 25 to 39 (CAREC member countries 2000). Given the incubation period, these individuals are likely to have contracted HIV during their years as youth, primarily as a result of unsafe sexual activity. Thus, in measuring the cost to society of youth behavior that results in HIV/AIDS, both the youth themselves and those who contracted HIV during youth should be considered.

The financial costs attributable to HIV/AIDS vary because there is no cure. Instead, costs may simply be incurred from treating other illnesses that afflict an individual with AIDS, estimated as US$200 per year per AIDS patient in Jamaica, for example, to the full "cocktail" that may cost $7,000 per patient per year (World Bank 2000a). Table 5-5 shows the per capita financial costs of HIV/AIDS programs, where the costs are a transfer from the whole population to those who require treatment (because treatment of HIV/AIDS patients in the latter two categories is paid through taxes), ranges from US$11 to US$61 per year for basic care programs to a range of US$85 to US$212 per year for basic care and aggressive treatment. Providing aggressive treatment to all HIV/AIDS patients would require an increase in health spending of 27 percent (Bahamas) to 1,111 percent (Haiti). Although table 5-5 accrues to the whole population, not just youth, it suggests how costly prevention and care is for those who contract HIV while young.

Forgone labor market productivity, under the worst case scenario where no HIV/AIDS treatment is given, is as high as 0.5 percent of GDP. If all new AIDS patients do not receive any treatment and die within one year (a very liberal assumption because AIDS patients are treated in many countries and the World Bank's new HIV/AIDS lending programs will further spread prevention methods and treatments) the loss to productivity of new AIDS cases in one year is less than 0.1 percent for most countries in the sample (table 5-6). The total forgone benefit to society, and especially to the family and friends of the AIDS patient, is clearly much higher. When measuring the loss of labor productivity in the year 2000 for *all* AIDS patients since 1982, under the assumption that all

TABLE 5-5: PER CAPITA US$ COSTS OF HIV/AIDS AND PROGRAM COSTS AS A PROPORTION OF CURRENT HEALTH SPENDING (ANNUAL)

	Basic care program		Basic care + HEART (at $7,000)	
	Per capita cost	**Increase in per capita health expenditures (%)**	**Per capita cost**	**Increase in per capita health expenditures (%)**
Bahamas	$61	8	$212	27
Haití	$12	67	$200	1,111
Dominican Republic	$11	12	$113	124
Guyana	$16	36	$198	440
Jamaica	$11	7	$85	57
Trinidad and Tobago	$12	6	$87	44

Source: World Bank 2000a.

men and half of the women would have been in the labor force (a safe assumption because the illness primarily affects people in their productive years), the loss to GDP in 2000 due to youth-contracted HIV since 1982 ranges from 0.1 to 0.37 percent of GDP.

Private economic costs: The forgone earnings given in table 5-6 largely accrue to the family of the income earner who died prematurely. Because a large portion of earnings of the individual would have been shared with the household, if the person passes away, a part of this is simply lost because other household members will not compensate for the full amount. Other private costs, which are less measurable, include:

- *Nonmonetary contributions to households in which the primary breadwinner or caregiver contracts HIV:* Among youth who contract HIV, most will have families by the time of onset

TABLE 5-6: FORGONE ECONOMIC OUTPUT DUE TO AIDS DEATHS

	Forgone output due to AIDS deaths in 2000		Forgone output in 2000 due to all AIDS deaths since 1982	
	Local currency, in thousands	**As % of GDP**	**Local currency, in thousands**	**As % of GDP**
Antigua and Barbuda	1,32.3	0.0074	1,092.0	0.061
Bahamas	1,668.8	0.037	16,496.9	0.37
Barbados	8,591.3	0.17	6,443.5	0.13
Dominican Republic	13,187.0	0.0041	139,680.6	0.043
Guyana	5,110.0	0.0044	132,890.0	0.12
Jamaica	69,350.0	0.022	316,407.5	0.099
St. Kitts and Nevis	791.4	0.089	593.6	0.067
St. Lucia	13.4	0.0007	675.1	0.036
Suriname	8,740.2	0.0025	139,843.2	0.040
Trinidad and Tobago	9,158.8	0.023	83,155.9	0.21

Note: Only those countries that reported wages were included in the calculations.

Source: ILO unemployment and wage data; Joint United Nations Programme on HIV/AIDS (UNAIDS) HIV/AIDS rates by age, 1982–2000.

of AIDS. When a young household member dies, his or her family suffers greatly as a result of the loss of income, the additional burden on the remaining partner and children, and the emotional costs to the household.

▪ *Loss of returns to the family from private investment in the individual:* Forgone returns to private investments are also a casualty of AIDS-related deaths. Parents and communities invest in their young people by providing resources for childrearing and human capital accumulation, with the expectation that the child or youth will give back to his or her community. Premature death from AIDS-related illnesses will necessarily eliminate the return on this investment, leading to parents who are less secure in their old age and communities that are less developed and secure.

Social economic costs: The measurement of the social economic costs of HIV infection of youth include the following items:

▪ *Loss of returns from state investment in the individual in terms of tax revenue:* Forgone GDP overestimates the cost to the state of AIDS deaths. Instead, the financial loss to the state is in terms of the forgone return to the state's investment in the individual before his or her death. Given the gestation period of HIV, many youth who contract the illness will have completed their (often) state-sponsored education and are just beginning their productive lives, in which they will "return" to the state by the payment of taxes and other nonpecuniary benefits. If the individual consumes from the state all that he or she pays in terms of taxes, the net social gain or loss is zero. However, because these are young individuals, who are likely to demand less from the state, they are likely to consume *less* than their share of taxes, thus creating a net loss for the state.

▪ *Forgone benefits of public investment in treatment of HIV/AIDS patients:* The (largely public) costs of treating HIV/AIDS indicate that resources are directed away from other possible productive uses. Thus, the benefits from using the resources in this alternative program— such as drug prevention among youth, nutrition programs for children, and old-age benefits—are not realized, increasing the economic costs of the illness.

▪ *Infection of others:* A study of HIV in Honduras (World Bank 2002) estimates that each HIV infection results in the infection of 0.1 additional individuals through sexual contact. Additionally, children (ages 0 to 4 years) with HIV/AIDS make up 3 percent to 4 percent of all reported AIDS cases (CAREC member countries 2000). These children are most likely to have contracted the disease from their mothers. Thus, cost estimates here per individual with HIV have much wider consequences.

▪ *Orphans:* Most individuals who contract HIV while youth will be parents of young children when AIDS-related death occurs, leaving a generation of children with one parent or no parents. Estimates from PAHO suggest that since 1982, the number of orphans per AIDS-related death range from 0.1 in Barbados to 3.2 in Haiti (table 5-7). Orphans, whether cared

TABLE 5-7: ORPHANS WHOSE PARENTS DIED OF AIDS-RELATED ILLNESSES			
Country	Orphans whose parents died of AIDS-related causes	AIDS-related deaths	Orphans per AIDS-related death
Barbados	190	1,800	0.11
Dominican Republic	7,900	4,900	1.6
Haití	74,000	23,000	3.2
Jamaica	1,200	650	1.8
Trinidad and Tobago	930	530	1.7

Source: PAHO (1999).

for by the state or other family or community members, will accumulate less education over their lifetimes, have lower earnings, have a higher propensity to engage in criminal activity, be less healthy, be more likely to engage in child labor, and be socially excluded, all of which lead to a less happy, healthy, and productive next generation, which imposes private costs (less income, less integration with society, poorer health) and social costs (transfers directed toward these adults rather than others in need, less government tax revenue, higher crime costs).

▦ *Forgone nonmonetary contributions:* Individuals not only contribute taxes to the common good, they also help to build a society. Premature deaths of prime-aged men and women will deny their societies of the contributions that they would have made to culture, democracy, and society, costs that are difficult to quantify.

▦ *Underinvestment in future generations:* As HIV infection rates increase, the incentive to invest in the future generation decreases because the likelihood that they will survive to realize those investments is shrinking. The implications of this for society are enormous because those who do not succumb to HIV/AIDS will be less productive (in monetary and nonmonetary senses) members of society as a result of less human and social capital accumulation while they were young.

▦ *Social exclusion:* Those with HIV/AIDS are still commonly excluded from society, as are their families, resulting in fewer contributions enjoyed by society and the individual.

▦ *Lower costs to government expenditures:* Although young people who die of AIDS-related illnesses are likely to have been net contributors to the state during their productive years, they are also likely to have been net debtors later in their lifetimes. Thus, early death from the illness will decrease the demands on the state, thus lowering financial and economic costs.

In addition to the financial costs to the state and family of treating a person with HIV/AIDS, the economic cost to the individual, his or her family, future generations, and society is enormous. Existing data and measurement techniques do not allow us to closely estimate the costs, but even the lower bound estimates are astronomical.

Unemployment

Youth unemployment is more costly to society than adult unemployment because, in the case of youth, human capital accumulation is interrupted early in the work life. On average, youth unemployment is three times higher than adult unemployment (see chapter 3), thus leading to larger forgone productivity. However, unemployed youth, as discussed in chapter 4, are active in violence, substance abuse, and risky sexual behavior, so these costs from other behaviors correlated with (and possibly caused by) unemployment may also be considered a cost of unemployment.[49]

The forgone productivity due to an idle factor of production—youth unemployment—ranges from zero to more than 7 percent of GDP in various Caribbean countries. If youth unemployment were eliminated, the increase in GDP would range from 1.1 percent in Barbados, to 5.7 percent in Jamaica, where 2.6 percent is due to additional male labor and 3.1 percent is due to additional female labor (table 5-8). The addition to GDP in the other countries in the sample falls between these extremes.

Table 5-8 also presents the forgone output by youth if their unemployment rate were equal to the adult rate and if it were equal to the youth unemployment rate in the United States, an alternative job market for many Caribbean youth. These estimates suggest that if the unemployment rate of

---

49. Few studies show that unemployment causes individuals to engage in these risk-taking behaviors, though focus group interviews suggest that unemployment combined with other factors (such as social exclusion) may lead to violence or substance abuse. Thus, adding the costs of risky sexual behavior, crime and violence, or substance use to the total cost of unemployment may be premature until further research corroborates the causal relationship.

TABLE 5-8: HIGHER GDP (%) IF YOUTH UNEMPLOYMENT RATE IS LOWER, DEMAND ELASTICITY = −2[50]

	Zero youth unemployment		Youth unemployment equal to adult unemployment		Caribbean and U.S. youth unemployment rate equal	
	Boys	Girls	Boys	Girls	Boys	Girls
Antigua and Barbuda	1.14	0.50	0.80	0.35	0.60	0.26
Barbados	0.56	0.54	0.30	0.42	0.40	0.45
Dominican Republic	1.68	1.50	0.85	1.34	1.33	1.49
Guyana	1.17	0.85	0.84	0.76	0.71	0.67
Jamaica	2.60	3.14	1.45	2.69	2.07	2.89
Saint Lucia	2.18	1.73	1.28	1.29	1.95	1.63
Trinidad and Tobago	1.50	1.05	0.80	0.76	1.17	0.9

Source: ILO unemployment rates and wage data (see Table A3-3 (Appendix 3) for years; author's calculations.

youth were equal to that of adults, GDP would still be 0.7 to 4 percent higher. If it were the same as in the United States, GDP in the Caribbean region would be 0.8 to 5 percent higher (table 5-8).

Economic costs: The forgone earnings in table 5-8 largely reflect economic costs of unemployment to the individual. Additionally, a portion of those lost earnings is economic costs to the state in the form of forgone tax revenue (firm or export taxes). However, additional indirect costs, some of which are costly to reverse, are also imposed, including:

- *Lower future income:* Labor productivity is rewarded in the labor market. An unemployed individual is not accumulating human capital to increase his or her labor productivity while unemployed, and he or she may even lose existing skills during the job search process.[51] The stagnation or destruction of skills will result in lower earnings when the individual does find a job, having negative implications at the private level (well-being of self and family) and the public level (lower tax revenues).
- *Migration:* An absence of jobs results in migration to more dynamic labor markets. Despite the assumption that only the well-to-do migrate, focus group interviews reveal that migration is a reality for youth across all socioeconomic classes. This is a loss to society because investments in these young people are realized in other countries and they are not generating the nonpecuniary benefits in their home societies, but some of this may be recovered in the form of remittances. Migration may lead to family and community breakdown and a generation of barrel children, who have few opportunities to be productive citizens, to the detriment of themselves and their countries.
- *Underinvestment in future generations:* If jobs are scarce, parents either cannot afford to send their children to school or they choose not to make this investment because of low expected returns. Although data do not exist to corroborate this claim, it is an issue that is worth monitoring because of the future private and public costs associated with a less skilled population.

---

50. A demand elasticity of wages of −2 is applied because as employment is created, the wage rate should fall (Maloney and Arango 2003).

51. Although unemployed individuals may maintain their human capital by volunteering or attending job training programs, these activities are increasingly rare in the Caribbean region.

▓ *Social exclusion:* The fact of being unemployed is a type of social exclusion, but activity in illegal labor markets is an alternative that is chosen more often by youth, further excluding them from mainstream society.

▓ *Secondary costs from criminality, substance use:* Unemployment is correlated with other youth behaviors that impose costs on the individual and society

Financial costs: Although the financial costs of unemployment primarily accrue to the individual, there are social financial costs as well. An unemployed person may collect unemployment insurance (as in Barbados) or be more dependent on the state for social services because he or she cannot support him- or herself. These public costs are likely to be minimal, though, because young people are still dependent on their parents, so the costs are privately born by the families. However, direct costs to both the state and the individual are imposed by the behaviors that tend to be associated with unemployment, such as increased drug and alcohol use or crime and violence.

School Leaving

Early school desertion imposes a high cost on the Caribbean region. As discussed in previous chapters, school not only provides the human capital that can be sold in the labor market, it also is the source of more general education, such as social interactions, building social capital, and identifying guiding principles for one's life. The discussion in chapter 4 suggests that simply being in a school environment is largely a positive force. Thus, early school departure may not impose large direct costs on society (holding constant the other negative behaviors that school leavers tend to engage in) but also impose high indirect costs in the form of forgone labor earnings for the individual, lower tax revenues for the state, and secondary costs of the risk-taking youth behaviors that result from either having less education or not being in school at a young age.

The personal and economy-wide gains to a population with a postsecondary education are far greater than for those with only a primary or secondary education. The marginal lifetime earnings from a university education, relative to a secondary education, are represented in appendix 3.[52] The differences are large for men and women in all countries presented. However, the graph also shows that the benefit to lifetime earnings of a secondary school education, relative to only a primary school education, is not as distinct. First, the gap between the middle line and the bottom line—comparing secondary school education lifetime earnings to primary school education—is not as large as the comparison between secondary and postsecondary, implying that the net gains are not as large. Second, the marginal benefit to women seems to exceed that of men, because women in all countries receive a higher primary to secondary education than do men, though it may not emerge until late in their work life. Finally, for some Guyanese, Jamaican, and St. Lucian men, the lifetime earnings from a secondary school education do not differ from those from just a primary school education. This may reflect the inability of secondary school to prepare young people for the labor market: Perhaps all skills that are valuable to the labor market are learned during primary school, and skills learned while working as a teenager earn a higher premium in the labor market than do skills learned during secondary school.

The discounted lifetime cost of early school leaving in terms of forgone earnings at the individual level, which may also be understood as forgone GDP for the country, reaches into the hundreds of

---

52. The top line in each graph is the amount of earnings at each age that an individual with university education receives at each stage of his or her life. The second line is the total earnings of a person with a secondary school education, and the bottom line is the earnings per year of an individual with only a primary school education. The area between each line is the net benefits to lifetime earnings of the next higher level of education. An alternative measurement is to estimate returns to each level of education and use the coefficients from a linear regression to estimate earnings. The weakness of this approach is that it assumes that the returns to experience for each education level are constant, which is clearly not the case, as shown by the graphs. The graphs are used because education and experience are the primary explanatory variables in a Mincerian wage equation and all the information from these variables is captured in the graphs.

	Dominican Republic 1998	Guyana 1999	Jamaica 1997	St. Lucia 1995	Trinidad and Tobago 1992
Secondary					$5.2
Men	$27.4	—	$11.4	—	
Women	$16.9	$238.6	$20.6	$279.3	
University					$14.5
Men	$137.0	$660.6	$156.9	$420.4	
Women	$86.9	$1,036.3	$115.4	$1,562.7	

TABLE 5-9: NET DISCOUNTED LIFETIME EARNINGS RELATIVE TO PRIMARY SCHOOL PER SCHOOL LEAVER, 6 PERCENT DISCOUNT RATE (IN THOUSANDS OF US$)[56]

—Net difference in lifetime earnings is zero or negative.

Source: Household surveys for the first four countries; World Bank (2000b) for Trinidad and Tobago.

thousands of dollars *per individual*.[53] Table 5-9 shows the benefits of a secondary education in the Dominican Republic, Jamaica, and Trinidad and Tobago.[54] For example, in the Dominican Republic, the net lifetime earnings of secondary education relative to only primary education are US$27,400 for a boy and US$16,900 for a girl. This implies that the productive capacity of the economy is severely underused as a result of secondary school leaving. The benefit of postsecondary education is even more dramatic, where the net earnings (productivity) are in the millions of dollars, such as for Guyanese and St. Lucian girls.[55]

Economic costs: The estimates in table 5-9 can be interpreted as a conservative estimate of the private indirect costs of accumulating less education, but a fraction of the totals is an economic cost to society. A man or woman is giving up the additional happiness that may come from having more income, whether to spend on oneself or one's family. However, income and consumption are taxed, so tax revenues that would have accrued to the state are not collected as a result of the lower level of investment.

The value of forgone productivity is a clear underestimate of the total cost to the individual and society of education that is attributable to the importance of education in determining other

---

53. Because the marginal dollar earned by the young man or woman today is not equivalent to a dollar earned in the year 2045, at the end of the young person's work life, it is necessary to discount the net lifetime earnings to take into consideration the lower value that a dollar earned in 45 years has relative to one earned today. These discounted values are also useful in a cost-benefit analysis when considering whether or not to implement programs to lower school leaving.

54. The estimates assume that the wage elasticity of demand is zero.

55. This is an overestimate because it is unlikely that the economy could provide highly skilled jobs to a population with 100 percent university completion rates.

56. The discount rate is a proxy for the rate of time preference, interest rate, and savings rate. The rate of time preference differs by person because the poor tend to have a much higher rate of time preference; that is, a dollar in 45 years is worth much less than a dollar today as a result of the need to meet immediate consumption needs today. However, the social rate of time preference may be much lower. The difference between the social and private rate of time preference gives an incentive for governments to intervene in private decisions. For example, the discounted value of a higher education may be very low to a student from a poor family, who would greatly value the labor income that he or she brings into the family today. However, society sees the long-term benefits of this young person's labor market contributions over the future as well, so the benefit to staying in school is high. To bridge the difference, the state would intervene to either force or compensate the young person such that the private discount rate is more aligned with the social discount rate and the young person chooses the socially (and privately) optimal behavior.

behaviors, which themselves carry costs.[57] Chapter 4 suggests a negative correlation between school attendance and other risk-taking behaviors, and other studies suggest correlations among out-of-school youth and other risk-taking behaviors. For example:

- *Crime and violence:* Juvenile delinquency is correlated with lower levels of education (Barker and Fontes 1996). This may be due to the lower cost of engaging in risk-taking criminal activity (because job and well-being prospects are scarcer for the less educated [Eckstein and Wolpin 1999]), the positive social influence of mentors and peers in the school environment, or delinquency being the best income alternative for an individual with few marketable skills. The social and private costs of crime and violence are clearly detailed and discussed above, and their magnitude significantly increases the cost to the individual and society of less education.

- *Sexual behavior (fertility, STIs, HIV/AIDS):* Those with less schooling also are more prone to engagement in risky sexual activity. This may be due to the lower cost of participating in such activity (because the forgone earnings may be less for less educated individuals), an absence of resources—teachers, school nurses, counselors—to assist with these decisions, or an absence of reasoning, bargaining, or information about responsible sexual activity and the risks (and costs) associated with unsafe behavior. Conservative estimates of the private and public costs of adolescent pregnancy and HIV, given in the above sections, greatly increase the cost of limited education.

- *Substance use:* Those who are not in school are more likely to regularly use alcohol, tobacco, and illegal drugs (Barker 1995), all of which impose additional direct costs on society and on the individual, in the form of drug treatment programs and greater dependence on social programs, and indirect costs in the form of forgone income, forgone tax revenues, higher public health needs, and risk-taking sexual behavior (Rees, Argys, and Averett 2001), among other outcomes.

- *Employment:* More educated individuals have more job prospects and will earn higher income, leading to both greater private gains (through higher income, more job opportunities, and the well-being associated with them) and public gains—through greater tax revenues and less dependence on the public social welfare system.

- *Health care:* Those with less education also tend to have poorer health practices. This may be due to a lack of learning about health and care of oneself or to the poverty associated with less education that limits resources to care for one's health. The clear private costs are lower well-being and lower wages, and the public costs are both financial (higher demand on the public health care system) and economic (loss of benefits of the alternative use of health funds on others).

- *Social exclusion:* The expulsion of young people from the education system may have far-reaching mental health implications for the individual. These may discourage the person from participating actively in society, seeking out public assistance, or contributing to society, negatively affecting both the individual and society as a whole.

- *Democracy, volunteerism, and cultural expression:* Even when higher education is controlled for, it is correlated with cultural development, greater volunteerism, and a multitude of other social factors (Haveman and Wolf 1984). These nonmonetary benefits are estimated to be equal to the marginal value of additional education, thus doubling the estimated return to education.

---

57. Few studies clearly show a causal relationship between low education and the listed behaviors. Although education would reasonably affect the behaviors, it may be argued that unobserved factors, such as the propensity to engage in antisocial behaviors or a high discounting of contemporaneous behaviors, may be the source of both school leaving and other risk-taking behavior. If this were the case, then less education does not cause the other risk-taking behaviors, but instead it is simply correlated with it.

Despite the question of whether or not these behaviors can be fully attributed to education, they are likely to have some additional impacts. The estimates and discussion do give a general picture of the richness of human capital that could be even partly realized by investment in youth education.

Final Thoughts

Rough estimates show that losses to society from risky youth behaviors—in terms of both direct expenditures and forgone benefits of alternative uses of resources—reach into the billions of dollars. Even though the costs are not fully measured in this chapter as a result of missing data or difficulty in quantifying many costs, the dollar values clearly show that youth are a valuable input to the health of the economy and the country and that their engagement in risk-taking behavior does have costs far beyond the individual, impacting the youth's family, friends, and fellow citizens as well. Although the private costs exceed the social costs, which would suggest that individuals would work toward decreasing the incidence of youth risk-taking behavior, they do not. This is likely due to several factors, including that individuals do not fully internalize the costs or do not have the resources to attack the problem, or the sources of the problems are bigger than the individual. This presents two arguments for the involvement of government and the private sector (both businesses and NGOs) in addressing these problems: First, risk-taking youth behavior has high externalities on society, as measured by social financial and economic costs, and second, youth and their families cannot (or do not) address the problems on their own. However, we do not pretend that an easy solution or the resources are available to fully solve any of these problems. The next chapter addresses the potential role of government, NGOs, and the private sector.

6

YOUTH DEVELOPMENT POLICIES AND PROGRAMS

Over the years, concerns have grown over youth issues in the Caribbean region and the need to promote youth as active players in national development. Without exception, Caribbean governments have responded by establishing ministries or departments to coordinate youth development activities and most have put in place policies and related programs (Danns, Henry, and LaFleur 1997). Nongovernmental agencies, and to a more limited extent the private sector, have also stepped in and developed programs to work with youth and assist them in overcoming the issues they face. However, the proliferation of programs, the cross-cutting nature of youth issues, and the lack of systems to monitor and evaluate programs make it difficult to assess the effectiveness of these efforts. Given that many at-risk youth are out of school, unattached to institutions, and hard to find, there is the additional challenge of identifying the nature of the problems faced by these youth and designing programs to meet their needs.

This chapter looks at progress on youth policies in Caribbean countries, presents examples of public, nongovernmental, and private sector programs that respond to youth needs in the region, and briefly describes the involvement of international development organizations in youth development. The chapter further provides perspectives on youth policies and programs based on a review of the international literature.

Caribbean Youth Policies

Youth policy responses in Caribbean countries have varied considerably. As appendix table A4-1 illustrates, many countries have a youth-specific policy in place (the Bahamas, Belize, the Dominican Republic, Guyana), are in the process of revising their policies (Jamaica, St. Lucia), have a draft policy accepted at the cabinet level (St. Lucia), or have draft policies (Dominica, Grenada, Trinidad and Tobago). Barbados, Montserrat, and Antigua and Barbuda are the only nations that have not moved to develop a youth-specific policy. Since 1995, the CYP has been an important actor in promoting an adequate policy framework on youth development in the Caribbean region, and to this end has provided advice and technical assistance to countries on policy design and implementation (the CYP's activities are discussed later in this chapter).

Institutional arrangements, which influence the thematic thrust of the policies as well as working arrangements with other government agencies dealing with youth issues, also vary. Most Caribbean countries have placed their youth focal point in education ministries (Antigua and Barbuda, Barbados, Dominica, Haiti, Jamaica, St. Lucia, St. Vincent and the Grenadines, the Bahamas), whereas Suriname has given primary responsibility on youth to its housing ministry. Guyana and Trinidad and Tobago have specific youth ministries linked to sport and culture, and Grenada's focal point on youth is in the Ministry of Youth, Sports and Community Development. The Dominican Republic is the only country that has a youth-only secretariat. Furthermore, the scope of policies differs across Caribbean countries, with some nations (St. Vincent and the Grenadines, St. Lucia, and Guyana) having very broad goals, and others (Jamaica, Trinidad and Tobago, and Dominica) have very specific (and, in most cases, numerous) objectives corresponding to their stated goals. Jamaica's youth policy, its thematic priorities, and institutional arrangements are described in box 6-1.

BOX 6-1: YOUTH POLICY IN JAMAICA

Jamaica's National Youth Policy—approved in 1994—establishes the following goals: (a) to strengthen and expand education and training; (b) to improve work ethics and training and promote entrepreneurial skills; (c) to increase awareness of nutrition, STDs, sexual and reproductive health, hygiene and sanitation, substance abuse and unwarranted risk taking; (d) to prevent drug abuse; (e) to enhance recreation and leisure; (f) to improve attitudes and decrease anti-social behavior; and (g) to develop strategies for youth participation in decision-making and social and economic development. In 1996, the now defunct National Advisory Council on Youth was created to monitor and evaluate the implementation of the National Youth Policy and to advise the Government on matters relating to youth development, but the Council.

During the 1990s and up to the present, responsibility for youth ping-ponged from the Ministry of Local Government (MLG) to the Ministry of Education and Culture, to the MLG and back again to the Ministry of Education and Culture. Although formal responsibility for youth is now firmly vested within education, in reality both agencies share the responsibility for planning and implementation of youth policies and programs along with the Ministry of Health.

In 2000, the Social Development Commission, a statutory body under the MLG established a Youth Development Strategy for 2000 and beyond, which aims to achieve: (a) better coordination and integration of programs, services, and activities geared toward youth development through the establishment of a National Center for Youth Development; (b) more effective and sustainable mobilization of resources to fund youth development programs and activities through the mechanism of a National Youth Development Foundation; (d) better expansion of and support for successful youth development programs and activities; and (e) increased representation and participation of youth in decision-making through national youth umbrella organizations.

In November of 2000, the National Center for Youth Development (NCYD) was created as a Secretariat within the MLG. The NCYD, which is now a part of the Ministry of Education, Youth and Culture, is intended to be the vehicle for the coordination of all youth programs and services and to be the common meeting point for youth and the agencies and ministries that provide services to them. The Council's mandate is to work in partnership with NGOs, other state agencies and ministries and the private sector. The primary functions of the center are in the area of research and policy advice, program design and development, program coordination and monitoring, information dissemination, program funding. According to the CYP, which works closely with Commonwealth countries to implement their youth policies, the National Center has been an effective coordinating body at the national level.

In 2002, the youth focal point shifted back to the Ministry of Education and Culture. Jamaica's youth policy is currently under revision.

Source: Based on Blank (2000).

A well-formulated, youth-specific policy—no matter how good it looks—is not the panacea. Having capacity, information systems in place to identify the needs of youth, and the flexibility to tailor programs according to specific needs, as well as finding the right balance between coordination and implementation, are all important ingredients for dealing with a cross-cutting issue such as youth development.

The Dominican Republic is a case in point. The country's youth policy has been lauded within Latin America for its substance as well as the program implementation processes it establishes (Rodríguez 2000). In 2000, the country approved its General Youth Law (*Ley de Juventud* No. 49/2000) based on which the Secretariat of State for Youth was created. The law allocates a budget of 1 percent of the national budget for the youth secretariat, and it establishes a local Youth Initiatives Fund to be covered by 4 percent of municipal budgets (Rodríguez 2000). From 1999 to 2000, the Secretariat of State for Youth's budget tripled and was expected to increase 10-fold in 2000–01 (US$15 million) and further double in 2002–03.[58] But the youth secretariat is also facing the pitfalls of trying to implement its own programs. For example, it is putting in place a national scholarship program that threatens to consume all its resources and would compete with other public and private institutions with similar programs. The Dominican Republic would be wise to learn from the experience of Venezuela, which in 1977 created a Ministry of Youth. The ministry had strong political support and was well funded with petroleum dollars, but it was dissolved a decade later because of competition from other ministries responsible for education, health, and employment, as well as notorious inefficiency and lack of experience in the management of public programs (Rodríguez 2000).

By contrast, Barbados has no youth-specific policy but has the reputation of having the most effective public program on youth. This is due in part to the political will and commitment of policymakers. But it is also due to a well-designed, well-functioning program. The work of the Youth Affairs Division is grounded in youth status surveys conducted every five years, a school leavers tracking system, and research on youth in other thematic areas. The division also has the autonomy to tailor its programs. Another example of an effective program is that of Dominica, which currently only has a draft policy but has put in place an effective system of youth officers who work at the local and municipal levels.[59]

An important component of youth development involves having a strong voice for youth at the local level. This is the case in St. Lucia, which has a long history of voluntary youth organizations. Specifically, 162 youth organizations operating around the island under the umbrella of the National Youth Council keep the government on its toes.

Last, youth programs that have moved from a risk- or problem-based orientation to a youth development perspective are experiencing success. Programs have traditionally focused on providing youth with leisure and sport activities and promoting their participation in the provision of community services (Alexis 2000). Although these types of activities have nurtured strong and positive characteristics in young women and men and contributed to making youth well-adjusted, productive citizens, there is increasingly a shift toward youth as key actors in development processes of their societies (Alexis 2000). This means moving from seeing youth as passive recipients of programs and policies to understanding and fulfilling the needs of young people as citizens in relation to their societies and involving them in their nations' broad development processes.

---

58. It also establishes a Youth Institutional System *(Sistema Institutional de Juventud)* comprising all the main institutional actors responsible for implementing youth programs. It is also the only law of its kind in Latin America to have established budgetary resources for program implementation. The youth secretariat will be staffed with 1,000 people throughout the country and establish Youth Houses (*Casas de la Juventud*) in the country's 30 provinces.

59. Armstrong Alexis (Regional Director, CYP [Caribbean Centre], Commonwealth Secretariat), personal communication (2001).

Youth Services and Programs in the Caribbean Region

As noted previously, governments, NGOs, and, to a more limited extent, the private sector provide services to youth (see appendix tables A4-3, A4-4, and A4-5 for examples). Government typically addresses youth issues through education, social safety net programs, job training, family services, sports, and culture. NGOs are also active across sectors. For example, the NYC-Dominca has a database of 141 organizations that provide different services to young people (see appendix table A4-6 for a sampling).[60] These programs play an important role in addressing the needs of specific groups of at-risk youth, including street children, children in inner-city communities, teenaged mothers, young fathers, drug addicts, children with disabilities, and other special needs groups. However, evaluation data on the effectiveness of these different interventions are generally lacking. These organizations are also plagued by problems common to civil society organizations in other countries, including lack of staff, limited space for programs, scarce and uncertain funding sources, and limited administrative capacity. A brief description of the types of services made available is provided below by theme, drawing primarily on information from Jamaica (Blank 2000) and Trinidad and Tobago (World Bank 2000b).

Education

Problems associated with out-of-school youth and joblessness have sparked demand for educational reforms in the Caribbean region. In the Commonwealth Caribbean, a number of countries—the Bahamas, Barbados, the OECS countries, and Trinidad and Tobago—have responded by developing comprehensive reform approaches, whereas others—Belize, Guyana, Jamaica, and the Turks and Caicos Islands—have followed an approach directed at specific levels of the education system (Miller 1999). In the case of Trinidad and Tobago, for example, a comprehensive reform of the secondary education system aims to achieve universal access, convert double-shifted schools to single shifts, extend the amount of time spent in the classroom, and use a new, standard, five-year curriculum (World Bank 2000b). According to the recently released white paper on education, Jamaica's educational reform targets include five years of secondary education for all students entering grade 7 by 2003 and beyond and 5 percent annual improvement in the number of students passing English and mathematics in the Caribbean Examinations Council (CXC) (in relation to the total grade 11 sitting).[61] Although it is beyond the scope of this report to comment on the status of educational reform, an impact assessment of reforms in OECS countries carried out in late 2000 indicates a relatively high degree of success in implementing change at the early childhood and primary education levels, but a moderate to low degree of progress in harmonizing education systems, secondary education, terms and conditions of teachers, and education financing (Miller, Jules, and Thomas 2000).

It is important to note that, although limited, ministries of education often provide other educational programs in addition to their academic training. For example, Jamaica's Ministry of Education and Culture implements several programs for in-school youth, including guidance counseling programs; the Peace and Love in Schools program, which aims to promote nonviolent methods of conflict resolution; Health and Family Life Education Programs; and isolated initiatives, such as the Kingston Secondary School Drummers, that use music and the cultural arts to promote literacy, provide training, and reduce dropout among students. The Mico Youth Counseling Center offers day and evening programs for parents, children, and adolescents (in- or out-of-school) who have emotional and/or behavioral problems.

Training and Skills Development

Training and skills development is the focus of many programs directed at youth, given their high levels of unemployment. Several large youth training and employment programs in Trinidad and

---

60. PIOJ 1999.
61. http://www.moec.gov.jm/white_paper.htm.

Tobago reach a total of about 15,000 youth annually at a total cost of some TT$50 million (see appendix table A4-9). The most important ones include the Youth Training and Employment Partnership Program, a limited liability company established and funded by government; the Junior Life Centers, Adolescent Development Community Life Centers, Skill Training Centers, and High Technology Centers operated by the NGO Service Volunteered for All (SERVOL); and the Youth Development and Apprenticeship Centers (former youth camps), run by the Ministry of Social and Community Development. Some of the training offered in the private sector is profit oriented, small scale, and unregulated by the government. More than 500 institutions are registered with the Ministry of Education as providers of technical and vocational training, but few have been through any process of accreditation or validation, making quality an issue of concern. Large companies also provide skills training to improve the human resources base for their respective industries.

The HEART Trust National Training Agency (NTA), a statutory body under the Ministry of Education, Youth and Culture, is responsible for coordinating Jamaica's technical and vocational education and training system and providing skills training. HEART/NTA supports a wide range of training-related activities (including residential and nonresidential). Total enrollment in HEART/NTA programs was equal to approximately 31,000 in 1999–2000; because approximately 70 percent of trainees were under age 24, the program reached about 10 to 15 percent of "unattached" youth. HEART also provides a six-month to one-year educational program aimed at raising the academic level (to at least the grade 9 level) of applicants who were unsuccessful in passing the entrance test for regular HEART/NTA programs.[62] During the 1990s, HEART Trust/NTA expanded nontraditional vocational training programs for youth, which aim to link training with work experience and develop positive work attitudes. Other public agencies involved in training programs include the Social Development Commission, which implements the Special Training and Employment Program.[63]

Limited evidence from evaluations carried out in Trinidad and Tobago indicates that training is generally useful but meets market demands only to a certain degree. Some indicators of success include requests from private sector industrial and business employers as well as state agencies and NGOs for the customization of its integrated training package, high participation by vulnerable groups, and strong demand by clients. Several tracer studies have demonstrated positive effects of technical training on beneficiary employment rates, earnings, rates of self-employment, labor force participation, pursuit of further studies, literacy and numeracy, and character (for example, motivation and attitude). SERVOL graduates have also fared well, with studies showing 41 percent fully employed, 27 percent employed part-time and two percent self-employed.

Social Protection

Across the Caribbean region, several social safety net programs target young people. In Jamaica, for example, programs amounting to an annual expenditure of about US$33 million include school meals, school fee assistance, grants to tertiary education students, welfare programs (including food stamps), and economic and social assistance (see appendix table A4-8). However, questions have been raised about the effectiveness of some social protection programs directed at youth. For example, according to the World Bank (2000b), the Trinidad and Tobago Public Assistance Program demonstrates inefficiencies, such as lax application of eligibility criteria and duplication of benefits, which result in disincentive to enter the labor market, as well as targeting problems.

---

62. Enrollment in the regular HEART/NTA programs requires that applicants be age 17 or older and pass an entrance test set at the grade 9 level of education.

63. The programs help youth acquire marketable skills; encourage attitude change and personal development among out-of-school youth, aged 18 and older, who are unskilled and unemployed; and channel their participants into skills training programs in HEART/NTA institutions or community colleges.

Microenterprise Development

Although fewer in number, some youth programs support entrepreneurship and business development. The Jamaican government facilitates access to microenterprise credit among young people
through the Micro Investment Development Agency, which initially targeted disadvantaged people
between the ages of 18 and 25. However, youth participation rates have been disappointingly low
(about 10 percent of the total potential beneficiaries). In a similar experience, the Community
Development Fund established by the Social Development Commission initially focused on youth
as the target group, but did not succeed in obtaining many clients among youth.[64] Junior Achievement, a program funded by the private sector firm Hewlett Packard and operating in St. Lucia,
however, is reportedly experiencing success. The Barbados Youth Business Trust, an NGO with
similar objectives, is also showing promise. Both programs teach entrepreneurship, economic self-
determination, and business skills development in schools and focus on making youth self-sufficient
in job creation. Last, the Commonwealth Youth Credit Initiative, which was approved by the
Commonwealth Heads of Government, is a regional scheme that was created to respond to youth
unemployment across the Commonwealth.

Family and Youth Services

Many Caribbean governments support family and youth services, although these programs tend to be
poorly funded and weak. The Trinidad and Tobago government operates or supports services for
youth who lack an appropriate family care environment or who have come into conflict with the law.
In addition to institutional care, which is relatively expensive, the government has created mechanisms such as nonmaterial family support and probation to allow the youth to remain within their
families when possible. However, the former type of intervention (institutionalization) has historically
suffered a variety of limitations—lack of qualified personnel, stigmatization of beneficiaries and difficult reintegration in the community, little family involvement, inadequate accommodation arrangements, and high costs—and the latter type of service (family support and probation) is severely
restricted in scope. In Jamaica, the Children's Services Division of the Ministry of Health has responsibility for abandoned, abused, and neglected children in need of care and protection, adolescents
with behavioral disorders, and youth offenders. There are four types of alternative care services for
children in need of care and protection: children's homes, foster care, places of safety, and adoption.

Community, Sports, and Leisure

"Youth work has traditionally been carried out as a means of providing young people with avenues
for collective leisure, exploration, talent development, and service to community" (Alexis 2000). This
orientation is reflected in both the location of youth issues within the public structure and programming. In St. Lucia, for example, youth work is located within the Ministry of Education but covered
by the Department of Youth and Sport. Youth initiatives supported by the department are thus
linked to sport and sporting facilities. In Trinidad and Tobago, youth-serving organizations have also
relied on sports as well as recreational and cultural activities to engage youth and promote positive
behaviors. Both the government—through the Ministry of Sport and Youth Affairs and the Ministry
of Social and Community Development—and the private and voluntary sectors have supported these
types of initiatives, and although they succeed to some extent in occupying youth's idle time and
contribute to socialization, they have limited potential to transfer useful skills. In this regard, the
organizations could take greater advantage of the ability of sports and culture to attract at-risk youth
by creating links to other services (for example, alternative education and skills training).

---

64. In response to these experiences and with the hope of making self-employment a viable alternative for
disadvantaged youth, HEART Trust/NTA recently modified its program curricula to include entrepreneurial
skills training as a requisite part of all of its training programs. To expand the number of persons able to teach
entrepreneurial skills, HEART Trust/NTA has provided training for trainers. The impact of these initiatives is
not known at this point.

In Jamaica, the Social Development Commission and the Jamaica Constabulary provide support to more than 1,200 youth clubs with over 25,000 members. Parents who are poor reportedly say that youth clubs have a positive impact on youth, particularly in rural areas.[65] Additionally, the Social Development Commission, Insport, the Sports Development Foundation, and private companies provide support for a program of sports infrastructure and community competitions in basketball, football, cricket, netball, track and field, and swimming. More than 300 communities participate island wide, and more than 200,000 persons participate in Insport youth and community club–level football, athletics, cricket, and netball activities alone.

Art, theater, and other cultural activities are increasingly used as vehicles to reach youth and deliver messages on youth development. For example, the Ashe Performing Arts Ensemble in Jamaica uses theater to convey messages on self-esteem and personal development, sexual and reproductive health, and parenting. Through workshops and performances, the NGO reaches inner-city youth between the ages of 10 and 24 years and parents of all ages.

National Youth Services
National Youth Services, which are organizations in which youth volunteers provide services in poor communities, are active in countries such as Barbados and Jamaica. The Jamaica National Youth Service, for example, a statutory organization under the auspices of the Ministry of Local Government (MLG), targets youth between the ages of 17 and 24 who are out of school and unemployed. Through "resocialization" and the development of appropriate work attitudes, the program aims to provide a bridge from school to career. Recruits are given one month of a core curriculum that stresses personal development and socialization, followed by eight months of work. National Youth Service workers are then assigned as teaching aides, community health workers and early childhood caregivers, or placed in the Cadet Corps and in the information technology sector. The program served approximately 1,600 young people in 1999–2000. It recruits young people who did well in secondary school—that is, those who completed grade 11 and passed four CXC subjects.

National Youth Councils
National Youth Councils (NYCs) are umbrella organizations or youth volunteer NGOs that provide services in their respective communities. The councils operate in Belize, Grenada, Guyana, Jamaica, St. Lucia, St. Vincent and the Grenadines, and Trinidad and Tobago. The St. Vincent and the Grenadines NYC, for example, was established in 1966 and has a membership of 57 member associations and clubs supported by dues, fees, and some limited public and international funding. St. Lucia's NYC, which is reportedly the strongest council in the Caribbean region, is a grouping of 162 youth organizations from St. Lucia's 18 branches. Seventeen of these branches are community based and distributed across the island, and the other branch comprises student councils from schools around the island. According to the St. Lucia Council, its biggest concern at this time is financial sustainability, given declining international resources, difficulties with attracting and employing required personnel, and the increasing dominance of individualism within the fabric of St. Lucian society, which discourages voluntarism. Given that they are often dependent on donor resources, the nature of their activities has changed somewhat as the councils have tailored their work around donor priorities (e.g., HIV/AIDS, mentoring, and job preparation).

NYCs provide an opportunity for youth to develop leadership skills. For example, several St. Lucian national and international leaders at one time served in the directive body of the St. Lucia NYC. See box 6-2 on a historical and future perspective of NYCs in the Caribbean region.

---

65. World Bank cited in Blank 2000.

BOX 6-2: PERSPECTIVES ON NATIONAL YOUTH COUNCILS IN THE CARIBBEAN

"National Youth Councils have been seen as significant youth structures for the expression of youth views and for taking the desires of youth to the corridors of power and decision making. NYCs have a relative long history in the region. As far back as the 1950s, young people sought to develop structures for addressing youth issues and issues of national development from the perspective of youth. The establishment of National Youth Councils was seen as an approach that would create avenues for young people. The Councils were formed with an interest to advocate on behalf of youth. They were guided strictly by youth and were often in stark opposition to governments and other agencies that maintained a paternalistic relationship with youth.

While youth interest in National Youth Councils reached its peak in the 1980s, the period of the sixties and seventies was one of political ferment in the region. Young activists were sufficiently sensitized to the political and developmental issues, which guided public opinion and policy at the time. As young people they thought it their responsibility to posit youth views on current issues. National youth leaders emerged, not because they were provided with opportunities but because they created opportunities to voice the concerns of their peers.

Significantly, very few of the National Youth Councils in the Caribbean were affiliated to the partisan political structures of the countries. The forthrightness of their leaders often placed them in stark opposition to the political status quo. However, their soundness, articulate expressions and strong personalities made them potential targets of the recruitment into political parties, which many of them pursued successfully.

It must be understood that National Youth Councils are youth structures established by youth to serve the interest of youth. They ought not to be the youth voice of any established structure working with youth. It is essential for NYCs to be independent of all external forces, working collaboratively with them but maintaining its autonomy. Through an NYC, structures working with youth should receive the perspective of youth. They should not dictate but should be dictated by the NYCs. The young people must desire to maintain that level of autonomy and independence."

Source: Alexis (2000).

Regional Programs
Commonwealth Youth Programme
The CYP is the youth department of the Commonwealth Secretariat that carries out decisions made by Commonwealth Heads of Government. Operating out of a regional office in Guyana and having covered the Commonwealth Caribbean since 1974, the CYP has 18 member countries. The CYP's main activities include training and empowering youth workers, providing technical assistance to governments on developing and implementing youth programs, supporting the economic enfranchisement of youth, and acting as a regional repository of information on youth in the Caribbean. Commonwealth governments provide the bulk of funding. But more recently, the CYP has collaborated with the United Nations Development Programme (UNDP), UNICEF, UNAIDS, and other partners. According to CYP staff, funding conditionalities have changed considerably over the years, having been more flexible in the past. At present, funding tends to be earmarked according to donor priorities, such as HIV/AIDS.

Caribbean Federation of Youth
The Caribbean Federation of Youth, which is based in St. Vincent and the Grenadines, was formed to act as a representative body for youth organizations in the Caribbean region and address problems faced by youth at the subregional and international levels. The federation's mandate is to coordinate the work of national youth organizations in the Caribbean region, assist them in policy formulation and management practices, and strengthen the integration process of Caribbean youth through networking, information sharing, and youth exchanges. The federation operates through the direct support of NYCs, which are responsible for implementing the federation's work at the national levels.

CARICOM

Led by its Commission for Human and Social Development (COSHSOD), CARICOM has recently become active in the area of youth development and has since worked hard to place youth issues on the regional agenda. Specifically, it established a Regional Strategy for Youth Development, which represents a framework for facilitating youth initiatives at the national level.[66] The strategy includes the following targets over the 2001–06 period: (a) all countries should have a youth statistical database and collect and analyze quantitative and qualitative data by 2003; (b) all countries should have systems for training and educating youth workers, and they should have begun to democratize and decentralize the youth function by 2003; (c) all countries should have NYCs operating and delivering services to youth by 2003; (d) all countries should have established mechanisms to provide youth with a voice in public policymaking by 2002; (e) all countries should have begun to implement intersectoral, community-based programs promoting economic participation, poverty reduction, sustainable livelihoods, and healthy families, communities, and nations by 2003; and (f) in terms of promoting adolescent health, all countries should have begun to implement community-based projects aimed at raising awareness, changing behavior, and empowering youth people to educate and counsel their peers by 2002.[67] CARICOM's other efforts include a Youth Ambassadors program, staging of model CARICOM conferences, and support for cooperative initiatives, such as the Australian Caribbean Community Sport Development Program.

International Development Organizations

International development organizations are active in youth development to varying degrees, with UNICEF playing a leading role due to its mandate on children and adolescents (see appendix 4, table A4-10). Working at the regional, national, and local levels, UNICEF organizes activities around the life cycle through three types of programs: early childhood development (0 to 8 years), adolescent development and participation (9 to 18 years), and social policy and special care protection. Types of programs supported by UNICEF in OECS countries, for example, include health and family education (using the classroom as the primary medium for transmission of messages), HIV/AIDS (peer training in partnership with the Red Cross), and youth empowerment (capacity building of NYCs). In the case of Jamaica, the UNICEF strategy is to promote cross-institutional collaboration in youth development through community-level, multipurpose hubs that provide integrated services to adolescents (UNICEF 2002).

Other international organizations that support youth development include the UNDP, which mainstreams youth work throughout its programs (reform of classroom culture, entrepreneurship, social policy development, community development, and information technology); PAHO, which supports integrated youth development programs;[68] The United Nations Population Fund (UNFPA), which funds adolescent reproductive and sexual health programs; the ILO, which funds work on child labor and job preparation; the European Commission, which addresses youth development through education and health projects;[69] the Canadian International Development Agency (CIDA), which supports youth development through a small grants program and an education project that addresses teacher quality and violence and discipline in schools; the U.S. Agency for International Development (USAID), which supports HIV/AIDS

---

66. www.caricom.org/archives/cohod/youth/youthdev.htm.

67. Key youth initiatives organized by CARICOM and its partners include (a) the Caribbean Youth Explosion 2000, which resulted in resolutions related to empowerment, representation, health, and rights of the child; and (b) meetings of directors of youth services in CARICOM, on which the CARICOM Regional Strategy for Youth Development was based.

68. Current PAHO initiatives in the case of OECS countries, for example, are in the areas of tobacco use, HIV/AIDS, mental health promotion, and health and family education.

69. European Commission activities include technical and vocational training, education sector reform (programmatic as well as project, with a push toward the former), institutional strengthening of community colleges, social investment funds, drug programs, and education and health infrastructure projects.

programs, community-based life skills and other training for at-risk youth, and parenting programs; and the U.K. Department for International Development (DFID), which, although not
supporting youth-specific projects, promotes youth development through education reform
(access to and quality of postprimary education) and eradication of drugs and urban poverty and
violence (in Jamaica).[70]

Youth Policies and Programs: The International Context
Global Policy Framework
Approved in 1995, the U.N. World Program of Action for Youth provides a global framework
for youth development. It identified 10 priority areas for action (to be carried out in two stages,
up to the year 2000, and from 2001 to 2010): education, work, hunger and poverty, health,
environment, drug use, juvenile delinquency, recreation, gender (girls and female adolescents),
and participation.[71] By 2000, according to a progress report on Latin America and the Caribbean,
of the 34 LAC countries, 27 had formulated a national youth policy, 30 had established a
national coordination mechanism for youth issues, and 16 had implemented a national action
plan for youth.[72]

Effectiveness of Youth Policies
Worldwide, there is a dearth of information on the nature and effectiveness of youth policies, due
most probably to the fact that youth development is a new and emerging field. Based on research
in the United States, Hahn (2002) notes that policy development in youth issues is new, underdeveloped, and uneven across states in that country. He further identifies the following weaknesses
related to youth policy, many of which most probably also apply to Caribbean countries:

- Youth policy remains largely a set of categorical, deficit-oriented funding streams, each with
  its own fiscal calendar, targeting provisions, performance standards, and the like.[73]
- Youth policies tend to lack age specificity.
- Youth policies tend to be all encompassing and fail to confront tough policy choices and
  prioritize target groups and issues.
- Policies tend to overlook the need to support the organizational needs of youth development service providers (e.g., in financial controls, organizational development, human
  resources development, planning and development, etc.).
- Confusion exists over the institution that should dominate the youth development field
  (education, child development, criminal justice, health, local or municipal agencies, culture
  and sport, etc.).

BOX 6-3: COST BENEFIT ANALYSIS OF PROGRAMS TO REDUCE TEEN CRIME

A study examining the cost effectiveness of different programs to reduce serious crimes in California found
that graduation incentives for high school youth were the most cost effective at about US$4,000 per crime;
followed by parent-training interventions at US$6,500 per serious crime and US$14,000 per crime presented
in the case of delinquent supervision. All three compare favorably to the high cost alternative of incarceration
(Greenwood et al. 1996).

---

70. Also noteworthy are the United Nations Educational, Scientific, and Cultural Organization's
(UNESCO) youth programs in LAC, which support youth forums, formal education, and the Infoyouth
Network (Pilotti 2002).
71. The Economic Commission for Latin America and the Caribbean (ECLAC) assists in the implementation of the action plan by holding regional meetings and preparing studies and reports on youth.
72. Secretary General 2001, cited in Pilotti 2002.
73. Deficit-oriented funding streams refer to funding that is directed at addressing youth problems
(or deficits) rather than focusing on the assets that youth possess.

▓ Many policy activities are in information, training, and collaboration; much less support exists for tangible program services, especially youth development programs that are comprehensive and long term.

Lessons from Youth Programs

Studies and evaluations of youth programs tend to be descriptive rather than presenting a critical analysis of program effectiveness, including their cost-benefits and so forth (Hahn 2002). Moreover, evaluations that have been carried out have been limited to single services or limited, short-term interventions rather than examining comprehensive youth development programs (Hahn 2000). However, according to James (1997, 1999), basic principles that underpin successful programs based on evaluations of approximately 100 youth programs in the United States include

(a) High-quality implementation, including ample start-up time; clear communication of goals; sufficient, timely, and sustained resources; strong leadership from the federal, state, or local levels; staff development; and the use of data to improve performance.
(b) Caring, knowledgeable adults, including parents, teachers, counselors, mentors, case workers, community members, program directors, or other trained individuals who understand and care deeply about youth, provide youth with significant time and attention, and provide support to youth over the long term.
(c) High standards and expectations, which means guiding the behaviors of youth, challenging their behaviors, and insisting on the personal responsibility and accountability of youth.
(d) A sense of community, including creating an internal feeling of community and family-like settings for young people.
(e) A holistic, comprehensive, multidimensional approach to working with youth that focuses on the individual and provides a range of protective factors rather than emphasizing one negative behavior.
(f) A focus on youth as assets, rather than on youth "deficits"—for example, service learning and community service programs give youth the opportunities to demonstrate to themselves, their parents, and their communities that they are able to contribute to society in positive ways.
(g) Guidance and connectedness to the workplace, including connections to jobs and employers, encouragement to pursue and succeed at work, and supports that extend beyond job placement (e.g., job coaches and mentors, structured opportunities to learn on the job, etc.).

Furthermore, based on rigorous analytical work of 49 programs, James (1997) found the that

(a) well-conducted mentoring programs, which are relatively cost-effective, can delay the onset of drug and alcohol usage among youth and boost school retention and performance;
(b) programs that stick steadfastly with at-risk youth through their high school years can have strong positive effects on graduation and college attendance rates (e.g., the Quantum Opportunity Program); and
(c) programs that lift employment and earnings for participants (e.g., young women on welfare) through occupational training that incorporates basic skills instruction and an open-exit policy allowing participants to judge for themselves when they are ready to take a job.

A review of recognized, international programs for at-risk youth was carried out by Barker and Fontes (1996) found the following:[74]

---

74. The analysis covered 23 programs (13 in primary prevention, 6 in secondary prevention, and 4 in tertiary education), selected on the basis of, among other things, the recognition of peer groups.

- Successful programs emphasized the completion of secondary education as a fundamental development need of youth (see box 6-3).
- Successful programs saw the need to pay youth to participate in vocational or training activities, given that at-risk youth often need immediate income support for their personal survival and to assist their families. But at-risk youth also required more long-term supports, such as life skills education, and long-term employment skills, such as job orientation.
- Programs to prepare youth for the self-employment sector were less effective because of the difficulties youth encounter in obtaining credit and technical and managerial skills to run a business.

As for institutional-related issues, Barker and Fontes (1996) found that few programs for at-risk youth that they analyzed maintained good information about cost-effectiveness or evaluated the impact and cost-benefit of their services. Other problems identified included (a) lack of staff training and long-term investment in personnel and, as a corollary, high staff turnover; (b) limited success in leveraging private sector funding and support; and (c) unstable funding sources. Programs that were found to be the most stable and successful had focused objectives, a clearly defined target population, tangible connections to the local community (including the local business sector), and instruments to assess needs and evaluate their efforts (see box 6-4 for guidelines on targeting at-risk youth).

Last, as pointed out in previous chapters, many youth do not take advantage of existing programs even when they do exist. The chief reason is that they no longer have faith in the system. Thus, a large population of at-risk youth generally does not make use of available programs. This situation suggests that if programs and services for youth are strengthened and expanded, they must be promoted in creative ways. As one youth leader from Jamaica put it, "The drug 'dons' [traffickers] promote themselves to the youth. We have to promote our programs too if we are to get the youth's attention" (Barker 1995). As countries move forward and evolve in addressing the problems faced by their youth, the hardest challenge will likely be reaching these excluded youth.

Final Thoughts
Youth Programs

In many ways, governments, NGOs, and, to a more limited extent, the private sector, have attempted to respond to the needs of youth in the Caribbean region, including low-income youth. Jamaica and

---

BOX 6-4: CLASSIFICATION OF YOUTH AT-RISK FOR TARGETING AND PROGRAMMING PURPOSES

Youth in Primary Risk are those youth who live in situations of disadvantage and poverty, are at-risk of leaving school or otherwise compromising their healthy development. These youth are still living with their families, and are attached to a school or another social institutions but are at-risk of losing their connections and suffering from a situation that jeopardizes their successful transition to adulthood and integration into society. This group faces general risks because of socio-economic circumstances but specific risk behaviors have yet to manifest themselves.

Youth in Secondary Risk are those youth who have moved from a general to a specific risk (e.g. by leaving school, working at an early age, being involved in a gang, facing physical or sexual abuse in the home, etc.) and are in danger of entering into a harmful situation. These youth have some connections to family or social institutions but these are weakening.

Youth in Tertiary Risk are those youth who are suffering the impact of particular situation (incarceration due to delinquency, drug dealing, adolescent motherhood) and have lost their connections to family, communities and social institutions. Services for this group include protective or intensive services, which are often residential-based.

Source: Barker and Fontes (1996)

Trinidad and Tobago, for example, have long histories of creative NGO and governmental efforts to assist at-risk youth in particular. St. Lucia's NYC is exemplary in creating an active voice for youth and ensuring that the government of St. Lucia is responsive to youth issues.

As a whole, it is difficult to know the impact of these programs. As pointed out by Alexis (2000), even though the Caribbean region has a solid track record of organized youth activity and numerous programs, it has neither the adequate systems nor the data and rigorous analysis to monitor the effectiveness of these programs. The cross-cutting nature of youth issues and the multitude of programs in place to address youth also make monitoring and evaluation a challenge. But problems related to measuring the impact of youth programs are not limited to the Caribbean region. Worldwide, very little exists in the way of impact evaluations of youth initiatives, which is likely attributable to the relatively young and underdeveloped nature of the youth development field.

Youth Policies

In terms of effective policy frameworks for youth, a youth-specific policy can be an effective tool for putting the youth issue firmly on the agenda of policymakers and creating ownership of youth development—particularly if the youth policy is approved through the representative wing of government (e.g., Parliament in the Commonwealth) rather than receiving only cabinet approval, as is the case of some of the youth policies. But clearly, a well-worded policy is not enough. As countries move to involving youth as active participants in development, programs with systems in place and the analytical rigor to identify the needs of youth and the flexibility to tailor programs accordingly will be more effective. As always with a cross-cutting issue, finding the right balance between coordination and implementation is another important element of an effective policy framework.

Unfortunately, as in the case of youth programs, little can be gleaned from international experiences because of the limited policy analysis that has taken place and the newness of the youth development area. Existing analysis of youth programs and policies, however, points to the need to carry out evaluations and cost-benefit analysis of programs; confront tough choices in terms of targeting and prioritizing issues to be addressed; define age specificity of services; provide longer-term, quality services; support programs that provide youth with access to caring, knowledgeable adults over the long term; and create incentives for private–public sector collaboration.

7

CONCLUSIONS AND
RECOMMENDATIONS

The House Is on Fire

Although the transitional period from childhood to adulthood is unquestionably a challenge for many, the majority of Caribbean youth make the transition unencumbered. Yet, as this report demonstrates, there are serious social and economic consequences associated with not addressing the minority group of youth who are at risk of negative behaviors or are suffering the impact of their negative circumstances—not only for the youth themselves and their families, but for society at large. As noted in *Time for Action, Report of the West Indian Commission* (1992), "While Caribbean Youth involved in crime and drugs or infected with AIDS remain a minority, it is the resources which must be diverted for their treatment and the loss of their creative potential and energies which make this minority of national, and indeed regional, concern."

As pointed out in writings from the Caribbean region, youth are "tomorrow's adults," "the pillars of tomorrow."[75] Indeed, investments in youth have potentially high payoffs at the individual, familial, and societal levels. Young people who contribute positively to society create positive externalities that improve the economic, cultural, and social environment for all. Policymakers and governments thus have a catalytic role in ensuring that youth are exposed to a full spectrum of opportunities to enable them to become productive, healthy adults.

The main risks facing Caribbean youth—teenage pregnancy, school leaving, unemployment, crime and violence, substance and drug abuse, and social exclusion—are not uncommon in developing as well as many developed countries. But as the study findings indicate, some risk outcomes are particular to the Caribbean region, for example:

> ▩ *Sexual and physical abuse is high in the Caribbean and socially accepted in many Caribbean countries.* Corporal punishment continues to be widespread in Caribbean schools and

---

75. Danns 1997; Alexis 2000.

homes, particularly among boys. And according to the nine-country CARICOM study, 1 in 10 school-going adolescents have been sexually abused. The high incidence among boys stands out in comparison to other countries. Even more noteworthy is the "disturbing pattern of cultural 'normalcy' in child and physical and sexual abuse" in the Caribbean region (Barrow 2001).

■ *The onset of sexual initiation in the Caribbean is the earliest in the world* (with the exception of Africa, where early sexual experiences take place within marriage). Early sexual debut is known to predispose young people to early pregnancy and HIV/AIDS and other STIs.

■ *The region has the highest incidence of HIV/AIDS outside Africa*—and youth are an at-risk group. Among other things, HIV/AIDS is linked to cultural values about sexuality that are particular to the Caribbean.

■ *The incidence of rage among young people is extremely high.* Forty percent of school-going CARICOM students reported feelings of rage. High rates of sexual abuse and physical abuse among children likely play out in rage among young people, which can affect their school performance and lead to violence.

■ *Youth unemployment is especially elevated in some Caribbean countries.* International comparisons indicate that Barbados, Trinidad and Tobago, the Dominican Republic, and Jamaica have high rates. Indeed, St. Lucia has the highest rate of unemployment in the Americas.

■ *In contrast to the United States, which has high levels of youth violence, the proportion of Caribbean adolescent males who carry firearms is extremely high.* Fully one-fifth of students had carried a weapon to school in the 30 days previous to the survey, and nearly as many had been in a fight using weapons. *Gang violence is also high in the Caribbean,* with 20 percent of male students and 12 percent of female students having belonged at one point to a gang.

■ Although data on drug use are scanty, anecdotal evidence suggests a *widespread social acceptance of alcohol and marijuana in some Caribbean countries,* among both in-school and out-of-school youth (Barker 1995). Out-of-school youth 13 to 19 years old are most at risk of substance abuse as well as drug dealing (Barker 1995). Further complicating the situation, the Caribbean is a major transshipment point for drugs entering the United States and Europe.

Rough estimates show that losses to society from risky youth behaviors such as teen pregnancy, school leaving, crime, and HIV/AIDS—in terms of both direct expenditures and forgone productivity—reach into the billions of dollars. For example, the total costs over the lifetime that are attributed to each cohort of adolescent mothers is estimated to be US$38 million in the case of Jamaica. Clearly, this calls for immediate attention and well-thought-out strategies and actions on the part of policy makers.

Youth Are Not the Problem

A clear message arising out of this report is that youth are not the problem but a product of their environments. For the most part, they react to the situation in which they find themselves. For a youth, drug dealing can be rational if no other forms of employment exist, his or her family needs money, and the drug lord protects the youth and gives him or her a sense of belonging. A young person may have few options if he or she has a mother who abandons him or her emotionally, a father who is not present, grades that are too low to continue in school, no or limited job options, and few economic resources. In the context of Jamaica's tight job market, for example, even rehabilitated youth who have turned their lives around have extremely limited options if they are from a stigmatized neighborhood (Addiction Alert, personal communication, April 6, 2002).

Evidence here suggests that the following factors underlie the behaviors and outcomes associated with youth in the Caribbean:

■ *Family:* The family is the strongest protective and risk factor for youth behavior and outcomes. It is protective in that family connectedness, appropriate levels of parental discipline, moral guidance, protection from dangers in the adult world, and economic support allow young people to acquire personal and social skills while young. Conversely, parental displays of negative behaviors (substance abuse, violence); physical, sexual, and emotional abuse by family members; and the absence of parental guidance and support are risk factors.

- *Schools:* Connectedness to schools is highly protective against all risky behaviors, including using drugs and alcohol and engaging in violence or sexual activity. For example, among school-going adolescents, the probability of sexual behavior falls by 30 percent for boys and 60 percent for girls if they are connected to schools. Conversely, the school system can have devastating effects on those youth with low academic achievement by not granting them a place in school and, as a corollary, making them feel socially excluded and "worthless."

- *Poverty:* Young people in disadvantaged situations are forced to find work and often have few options except informal sector work, drug trade, or prostitution. Poor parents—particularly those who are single parents—are more likely to be absent from the household, leaving youth and children unattended and unsupervised. Young girls in some countries—often at the encouragement of their mothers—will engage in opportunistic sex to relieve poverty and contribute to household income (Williams 2001). And childbearing is still used a strategy for gaining economic support in such countries as Jamaica. Last, the income inequality made obvious by the presence of drug dons, foreign tourists, and the media encourages the engagement of youth in "easy money" activities, including drugs and prostitution.

- *Gender:* Gender,[76] which is linked to family dynamics and formation, is a central risk factor in Caribbean societies. About 85 percent of children in Jamaica and St. Lucia are born out of wedlock. The absence of fathers in the lives of children (which dates back to colonialism, when men were not permitted to pay the role of father and spouse) is linked to contradictory societal norms that, on the one hand, encourage multifathering and sexual prowess but, on the other hand, only allow men to be fathers if they provide economic support to the children. Gender norms and values have important intergenerational effects in that the children of absent fathers are more likely to fare poorly in school. Men's inability to meet the expectation of being an economic provider also means that a large proportion of women need to raise children on their own, leading to greater levels of poverty and vulnerability among these women and their children. Moreover, the children of single mothers are more likely to go unsupervised and be exposed to negative peer groups that prey on children (e.g., gang leaders and others) and to adopt their illicit practices (crime, drug dealing, and prostitution).

As the above paragraph indicates and consistent with the international evidence, factors underlying negative youth behaviors and outcomes are highly interrelated. The empirical analysis of risk and protective factors carried out using the nine-country CARICOM data demonstrates the interconnectedness of family, school, and community risk and protective factors. Results here also show that changing any one of the risk factors will help to reduce negative outcomes.

Youth Programs Abound—but Are They Effective?

Available evidence suggests that much is being done in the area of youth development, with government and the NGO sector both active in different ways. Innovative private sector and private–public sector initiatives for youth also look promising. But limited information on the situation of youth themselves—particularly out-of-school youth who are unattached to formal institutions—and on the nature and effectiveness of the multitude of programs that exist makes evaluation and informed planning difficult. Further complicating matters is the cross-cutting nature of youth issues, which implies a need for effective coordination across institutional lines and is a challenge under the best of circumstances.

---

76. As defined previously, gender, in the context of risk or protective factors, refers to the values, customs, and behavioral norms that account for sexual differentiation in identity and behavior.

At the regional level, CARICOM's Regional Strategy for Youth Development represents an important framework for placing youth on the regional agenda. And the CYP has been a key actor in assisting Caribbean governments to develop and implement youth policies, as well as in building a cadre of youth who are qualified to work on youth issues.

Moving Forward—Youth Development Principles and Actions

The situation that many disadvantaged Caribbean youth find themselves in and the costs that at-risk youth behaviour imposes on society call for decisive action on the part of policymakers. And as the previous section indicates, the problem is not the youth themselves, but the familial, community, social, and economic environment in which youth live and operate. Thus, the challenge for policymakers is to facilitate a process and create an environment that maximize the protective factors while reducing the risk factors affecting youth. Going back to the conceptual framework at the beginning of the report suggests public action in two spheres: the macroenvironment—including the macroeconomy, public institutions (education, public health, judicial system), and socio-cultural norms and values, which among other things influence gender roles and relations, family structure and dynamics—and the microenvironment, including families, neighborhoods, communities, the faith community, local governments, and other community-based institutions.

Youth Development Principles

Building on available research and practice, this report puts forward a set of principles to guide youth development efforts in Caribbean states at both the macro- and microenvironment. These include (a) a life-cycle, age-specific approach; (b) selectivity and focus; (c) an asset-based approach; (d) comprehensive long-term supports for youth; and (e) intersectoral, integrated approaches.

A Life-Cycle, Age-Specific Approach

Following on the experiences of UNICEF and others, youth development should be part of a life-cycle approach to human development (UNICEF 2002, Ferber and Pittman 2002). As noted in this report, many at-risk youth behaviors as well as problems faced by young people result from sub-optimal experiences earlier in life. In addition to providing a "safe passage to adulthood," young people require "a good start in life" (UNICEF 2002). Youth development thus must be part of a larger human development effort that takes into account different stages of the life cycle and corollary needs at different development stages, and programs and policies must therefore be age specific. The Forum for Youth Development in the United States, for example, defines target age groups as early childhood (0- to 5-year-olds), elementary (6- to 10-year-olds), middle school (11- to 14-year-olds), high school (15- to 19-year-olds), and young adults (20- to 24-year-olds) (Ferber and Pittman 2002). The Government of Jamaica UNICEF Country Programme 2002–2006 organizes its activities into two age groups: early childhood development (0- to 8-year-olds) and adolescent development and participation (9- to 18-year-olds) (UNICEF 2002).

Selectivity and Focus

The reality of resource constraints implies the selectivity and prioritization of youth development interventions as well as efficient targeting. International experience also demonstrates that the most stable and successful youth development programs have focused objectives and a clearly defined target population. As previously noted, a classification system to define youth target groups and their needs is as follows: *youth at primary risk* (youth who live in situations of disadvantage and poverty and are at risk of leaving school or otherwise compromising their healthy development), *youth at secondary risk* (youth who have moved from a general to a specific risk and are in danger of entering into a harmful situation), and *youth at tertiary risk* (youth who are suffering the impact of particular situation and have lost their connections to family, communities, and social institutions).

An Assets-Based Approach
As research and practice indicate, youth development programs should center on youth as assets rather than on the problems or deficits of young people. For example, the Big Brothers and Big Sisters program in the United States is centered on the mentoring relationship rather than on eliminating drug and alcohol use, but it has been found to decrease this at-risk behavior among participants (James 1999). Similarly, the U.S.-based Teen Outreach Program is focused on engaging youth in community services but has been found to decrease teenage pregnancy significantly compared with comparison groups (James 1999). In addition to focusing on the positive assets of youth, programs also need to hold youth to high standards, which means guiding the behaviors of youth, challenging their behaviors, and insisting on their personal responsibility and accountability.

Comprehensive, Long-Term Supports for Youth
Youth and children need more than academic or vocational training; they require support to develop their social, moral, emotional, physical, and cognitive competencies.[77] Empirical analysis also shows that programs need to be longer term and stick tenaciously with youth to gain a young person's trust, commitment, and active participation.

Intersectoral, Integrated Services
The comprehensive needs of children and youth are best met through intersectoral coordination and collaboration as well as public–private sector involvement. Many countries and states have established interagency youth structures with the objective of planning, coordinating, monitoring, and, in some cases, funding youth development interventions. Others have moved beyond coordination and are experimenting with an integrated services model for youth development, which involves establishing a collaborative arrangement between service providers (governmental, nongovernmental, and private sector) and the communities in which youth and their families live. The government of Jamaica, for example, is working with UNICEF to apply an integrated services model for youth in four pilot parishes (UNICEF 2002). Colombia and Chile are also piloting the integrated services model for youth development at the neighborhood, community, and municipal levels. This integrated approach has the objective of (a) reforming the usually fragmented system of services and supports for youth and their families; (b) providing an integrated and comprehensive range of services for youth and their families; (c) increasing community participation in, ownership of, and control over local initiatives; and (d) increasing transparency. Providing integrated services is complex in that it involves systemic change, new governance structures, and long-term investments in community development and local level capacity building, but it has also been found to be more sustainable than past approaches.

Recommended Actions for Youth Development
Specific recommendations corresponding to the macro- and microenvironment follow. Because country conditions vary, not all recommendations apply to each country. As previously noted, programs and policies as well as specific actions must be context specific and should be based on the nature and acuteness of the youth issues faced by each country as well as the institutional context.

Reform the Education System and Maximize the Protective Effects of Schools
The education system—and its manifestation in the microenvironment, the local school—can be highly protective during adolescence and thus represents a key intervention point for policymakers.

---

77. Developmental areas defined by the U.S.-based Forum for Youth Development include (a) learning, that is, developing positive basic and applied academic attitudes skills and behaviors; (b) thriving, that is, developing physically healthy attitudes, skills, and behaviors; (c) connecting, that is, developing positive social attitudes, skills, and behaviors; (d) working, that is, developing positive vocational attitudes, skills, and behaviors; and (e) leading, that is, developing positive civic attitudes, skills, and behaviors (Ferber and Pittman 2002).

Schools represent more than academics and learning. They are a source of social interaction and socialization. Thus, efforts should be aimed at improving access and retention and the quality of education, as well as using schools as a mechanism for positive socialization and social change. Actions directed at improving the formal education system and the positive effects of schools would benefit youth generally as well as primary and secondary at-risk youth. Types of actions would include:

- increasing the number of physical spaces where lack of space is a constraint (e.g., St. Lucia, Jamaica);
- applying voucher programs along the lines of Mexico's PROGRESA, where financial deprivation and the direct costs of schooling (e.g., school fees, transportation) are the pivotal constraints or where the opportunity costs of going to school are high;
- reducing overcrowding by providing for a sufficient number of qualified teachers (Samms-Vaughan 2001);
- improving the quality of teachers by strengthening teacher training and increasing in-service training (Samms-Vaughan 2001);
- rethinking the rigid model of education inherited from the British, which clearly underserves a segment of the adolescent population (Experience from the United States indicates that holding students back, for the most part does not serve students well);
- reforming the school curriculum to include learning modules on life skills,[78] basic job skills,[79] and reproductive and sexual health:
- eliminating corporal punishment that constitutes abuse in schools but maintaining discipline and imposing boundaries, which is important in the development of youth;
- putting in place educational activities and school-based campaigns to change attitudes on violence and teach conflict resolution; and
- contributing to reducing sexual abuse and exploitation by institutionalizing permanent school-based information and education campaigns to teach children and adolescents the difference between healthy and unhealthy sexual relationships, as well as their rights and responsibilities to report sexually abusive and exploitative relationships.

Although attractive, full-service schools—which in countries such as the United States provide a range of recreational and extracurricular activities (including health services on-site)—are not inexpensive. Moreover, most Caribbean education systems already have a number of deficiencies that would take higher priority—for example, increasing the number of school places, reducing crowding, and improving the quality of teachers. Thus, at the risk of overburdening the school system and diverting precious resources away from basic reforms, this report suggests that schools develop partnerships with NGOs and community organizations to provide parallel extracurricular services for youth that serve to reinforce the life skills lessons learned in school as well as providing recreation and safe spaces for youth. Last, vocational education should be in partnership with the private sector, which is better suited to identify areas where a shortage of skilled workers exist and the specific skills required.

Upgrade the Public Health Care System
As in the case of schools, the public health care system has a central role to play in addressing a range of critical issues affecting adolescents, including accessibility to reproductive and sexual health services, addressing sexual and physical abuse, helping people deal with rage, and so forth.

---

78. A life skills curriculum includes communications, conflict resolution, decisionmaking and problem solving, developing effective and affective relationships, childrearing and parenting, and values and beliefs as they affect decisionmaking and choices.

79. Experience shows that youth need help looking for jobs, marketing their skills, preparing for job interviews, improving human interaction and communications, and building effective relationships on the job.

But to be effective, existing public health care service providers require new protocols, tools, and techniques to work with youth and their family members, including mental health approaches.[80] Medical and nursing school students and graduates also need to be trained in these new protocols. Indeed, a review of international health outreach and health promotion programs for at-risk youth found that many staff encountered difficulties in addressing issues such as adolescent sexuality because of their own value systems and conflicts (Barker and Fontes 1996). Protocols should take into account the need for confidentiality and the differentiated needs of male and female patients.

The nursing and medical professions should play a pivotal role in condemning unhealthy sexual practices among children and adolescents by lobbying to make this a public health issue. In the United States, the nursing and medical professions were central in creating public awareness of this social issue. Given that sexual abuse and exploitation are rooted in social and cultural values, the nursing and medical professionals can play an important role by showing that sexual abuse is unacceptable and, indeed, an issue of public health. Actions directed at improving the public health care system and the positive effects of schools would benefit youth generally, as well as primary and secondary at-risk youth.

Reform and Strengthen the Legal, Judicial and Policing Systems

The high incidence of sexual and physical abuse, crime and violence, gang violence, and substance abuse in the lives of adolescents points to the need for improvements in the legal, judicial, and policing systems of Caribbean countries. Most Caribbean countries have put in place laws against incest, child sexual abuse, and other forms of abuse (Le Franc 2001), but police and society generally turn a blind eye to these offenses. Other issues related to juvenile justice include the legal definition of "a child;" the age of criminal responsibility, arrest, trial (pre and post), and detention; the management of detention centers and children's homes, and noncustodial alternatives (Singh 2001). For example, in the Dominican Republic, laws protect minors younger than 18 years old from being arrested, legally processed, and going to jail, thus creating a perverse incentive for drug dealers to target adolescents in drug and other criminal activity (Luther, St. Ville, and Hasbún 2002). Researchers have also called attention to the appalling practices of juvenile justice in the Caribbean region and the imprisonment of child offenders owing to the lack of facilities for young delinquents (Singh 2001). Or, as in St. Lucia, abandoned children or those who have been removed from their parents' home share facilities with petty criminals, thus exposing children who are at risk to higher degrees of risk. Last, the high incidence of school-going males carrying weapons suggests issues related to the availability of firearms in the Caribbean. Some areas for intervention include:

- Improving juvenile justice by reviewing and harmonizing laws, establishing and strengthening family courts, training legal practitioners, modernizing the court system, and using alternative custodial sentences.
- Increasing weapons controls by making it more difficult for youth to obtain firearms and establishing disarmament policies. In the United States, schools have put in place disarmament policies; firearms are also banned at specific youth events (McAlister 1998). Countries such as Colombia reported a 20 percent decrease in death rates when laws were put in place to disarm the public (McAlister 1998).
- Reforming the police[81] by seeking to reduce police corruption, strengthening the accountability of police, and improving community relations,[82] which are seen as the most promising

---

80. Issues of rage, sexual abuse, and suicidal tendencies require new mental health protocols oriented to both victims and perpetrators—for the former, to help them overcome their trauma, and for the latter, to provide rehabilitative therapy (Rock 2001).

81. Unless otherwise stated, the section on policing is based on Neild (2001).

82. Improving community relations and police legitimacy has led to the public cooperating in the identification of suspects and witnesses, in the investigation of cases, and making cases based on witnesses and material evidence (Neild 2001).

approaches to improve police effectiveness.[83] Directed patrols in crime hotspots also appear to have a positive effect in reducing crime in high-risk areas.[84] Indeed, evidence suggests that the most effective long-term strategy for crime prevention includes changing both the style and the substance of policing practices, the latter referring to how respectfully police treat suspects and citizens (Sherman 1998, cited in Neild 2001). Experiences with community policing suggest that this mechanism can be effective in improving the perception of public safety and image of the police but not necessarily in reducing victimization rates (Buvinic and Morrison 2001). With respect to sexual violence among adolescents, governments must make the police accountable for investigating and prosecuting perpetrators.

Interventions in the area of the judiciary and policing would benefit the population at large but are likely to have a greater impact on the tertiary at-risk group.

Institutionalize a National-Level Adolescent Mentoring System

A third central policy area concerns building a national-level mentoring system, which would primarily benefit primary and secondary at-risk youth. Connectedness to an adult, any adult has been found to be the single most important protective factor of youth development. And in the United States, mentoring programs have been found to be the single most cost-effective mechanism for creating connectedness among at-risk adolescents. Effective mentoring programs are professionally run and involve one-on-one pairing of an adult with a child or adolescent (during the formative years) and the provision of necessary support to make the relationship effective. The mentor develops a relationship with the child or youth, works to build the child or youth's self-confidence and sense of belonging, and spends time with and provides guidance to him or her.

NGOs and the private sector have a central role in implementing and supporting mentoring programs. Some U.S. firms, for example, give employees four hours of paid leave per month for the purpose of mentoring. Within the Caribbean region, the Big Brothers Big Sisters International mentoring program is operating in Antigua and Barbuda, Barbados, the Cayman Islands, and Grenada.[85] Governments should thus provide the incentives to ensure that these programs operate effectively and have broad coverage.

Use the Media and Social Marketing

Communication and education campaigns and the mass media should be used to change norms and values related to the following key risk areas for youth: sexual abuse and exploitation, early sexual initiation, corporal punishment and physical abuse, and alcohol consumption and drug use. They can also be used to teach effective parenting skills, promote the participation of fathers in the rearing of their children, and reflect positive role models and images for youth. National communication campaigns that are goal- and process-oriented, audience-focused, and that use multiple channels of communication, can be effective in changing social norms and values and behaviors (Suárez and Quesada 1999). Although this report has not offered a comprehensive analysis of mass media in the Caribbean, it is clearly an area that warrants serious attention, especially as radio, film, and, especially, television become more influential in informing young peoples' social values.

---

83. Although the effect of policing in preventing crime is a subject of considerable debate, there is a consensus that the police force is a key institution in improving the prosecution of offenders and reducing the fear of crime.

84. Research indicates that measures to expand and increase the power of police forces is not only expensive but has limited effect. Moreover, expanding police powers poses the threat of increasing levels of violence, undermining democratic processes, and further eroding the confidence of the criminal justice system if there is no oversight from political and judicial authorities, communities, and civil society (Neild 2001). Other measures that have *not* been found to be effective include more rapid response to telephone calls, random patrolling, and increasing the number of reactive arrests (Neild 2001, Buvenic and Morrison 2001).

85. For more information, see http://www.bbbsi.org/.

Social marketing, which draws on commercial marketing principles, has been used as a highly effective tool worldwide to change social norms and behavior. Using vehicles such as mass media, social marketing has been used in meeting social objectives related to nutrition, family planning, and health (controlling drug use, smoking, use of seat belts, etc.). Social marketing can be used to broadly target the population or specific groups (e.g., mothers and fathers of primary at-risk youth).

Make Family and Fathers a Top Public Policy Issue
The family is one of the most important risk factors in the development of Caribbean youth, and it is thus a central entry point for public policy. As a first step, governments need to put family and fathers firmly on the public agenda to demonstrate the critical nature of the issue. Second, it must put in place incentives to make parents accountable for their children, through the legal system, tax breaks, and so forth. For example, parents need to be held responsible and prosecuted for sexual abuse and the sexual exploitation of their children. The education system, the public health system, and the media can also play a role in promoting healthy families and teaching fundamental parenting skills. For example, studies have shown that the levels of physical and sexual abuse are significantly reduced when parenting skills are taught after the birth of children and programs are family focused rather than child centered (Le Franc 2001). As for fathering, a number of Caribbean NGOs work actively on this issue. But as in the case of families and parenting, public policies should explicitly promote responsible fathering and access of fathers to their children.

The private sector can play a key role in promoting profamily work policies. To illustrate this point, private companies could provide parents—both mothers and fathers—with a specified number of hours of paid leave to attend parent-teacher meetings (e.g., two hours a month).

Strengthen Community and Neighborhood Supports for Youth
NGOs, local organizations, and churches in the Caribbean region, which provide a range of services to youth and their families, are a good alternative to public services. These organizations have the advantage of greater flexibility and capacity to adapt and innovate, as well as greater credibility because of their proximity to the people and communities they serve. Moreover, local organizations and NGOs are often the only source of support for youth in the tertiary at-risk category. Governments should therefore directly support these organizations. One alternative would be to establish a competitive, community-based youth fund to finance initiatives addressing youth issues. Criteria for selection could include effectiveness, innovation, and sustainability. For example, the Dominican Republic is currently setting up a $7 million fund to support early childhood development programs at the local level.[86] Given very limited evaluation data on the effectiveness of local youth initiatives, putting in place an effective monitoring and evaluation system would be a prerequisite for funding.

---

86. The selection committee comprises representatives from civil society, academics, community leaders, and so on, although the government of the Dominican Republic has overall oversight responsibilities.

Appendix I

METHODOLOGICAL
DESCRIPTION FOR CHAPTER 4

The evidence for chapter 4 is based on two studies commissioned by the World Bank: (1) qualitative data collection and analysis of the reasons why youth engage in risky behaviors and the implications and (2) quantitative data analysis to identify the risk and protective factors responsible for risky youth behavior. This appendix discusses the data and methodology behind the results from each study.

Qualitative Data Collection and Analysis

Qualitative data were collected in the Dominican Republic and St. Lucia in the period February to April 2002 by the Instituto Dominicano de Desarrollo Integral with the National Youth Council of St. Lucia. The data collection comprised two components: focus group discussions with youth and structured interviews.

Focus Groups

Twenty-six focus group discussions were conducted: 12 in the Dominican Republic and 14 in St. Lucia. Each group had 6 to 10 participants. Treatment and control groups of youth were interviewed. Adults were interviewed for purposes of triangulation and to get their own views. The participants of the focus groups were

Dominican Republic:

- urban young men aged 14 to 24 (two groups),
- rural young men aged 14 to 24 (two groups),
- urban young women aged 14 to 24 (two groups),
- rural young women aged 14 to 24 (two groups),
- rural adults and peers (one group),
- urban adults and peers (one group), and
- control groups aged 14 to 24 (one urban, one rural).

St. Lucia:

- urban young men aged 14 to 24 (two groups),
- rural young men aged 14 to 24 (two groups),
- urban young women aged 14 to 24 (two groups),
- rural young women aged 14 to 24 (two groups),
- rural adults and peers (two groups),
- urban adults and peers (two groups), and
- control groups aged 14 to 24 (one urban, one rural).

The criteria for the selection of the treatment groups required that the young person had at least one of the following characteristics:

- belongs to a lower socioeconomic population (including drug pushers, gang leaders, and persons who rely on the sex trade),
- has abandoned school more than a year before the time of the interview,
- is not employed or working in a family business (except for those "employed" in criminal behavior),
- is not an active member of a formal community group or does not participate frequently in its activities (could be affiliated with informal youth groups: gangs or groups that gather for informal leisure activities), or
- is sexually active.

The control group participants did not have any of the above characteristics.

A two-step process was used to recruit the focus group participants in the Dominican Republic. First, the consultant selected the neighborhoods and communities that would participate in the study, using the sociodemographic studies available on slums in the National District. Similar areas were chosen for the urban zone on the basis of socioeconomic status, with an effort to control for differences in poverty levels. All the neighborhoods selected were poor, where poverty is reflected in all its aspects. Rural communities were chosen from zones with similar characteristics to the urban communities. Second, once the poverty-stricken urban zones in Herrera, Los Alcarrizos, and Capotillo were selected, as well as the rural communities such as Elias Piña and Bayaguana, the consultant recruited young participants through neighborhood leaders who personally made the contacts with participating candidates. Money for transportation was given to all the participants.

In St. Lucia, the recruitment process was done in coordination with the National Youth Council. Various government agencies and nongovernmental organizations (NGOs) assisted in identifying the target groups. The selected participants represented a broad cross-section of St. Lucian youth and adults, both in terms of territory and the composition of the groups.

Professional facilitators were used in both countries. The sessions lasted approximately one hour and a half. A session was composed of (a) administrative issues (objectives, clear statement of the ethical issues, request of verbal authorization to participate, confidentiality of the discussions, and respect for one another's' views), (b) a warm-up session, (c) conversations based on a semi-structured interview guide, and (d) a closing session and next steps.

Structured Interviews

Twelve one-on-one interviews were held with key informants on youth issues in the Dominican Republic, and 25 were held in St. Lucia. The interviewees included men and women who work with youth from government, civil society, and the private sector. The individuals interviewed ranged from a prime minister to leaders of community youth programs to religious figures. Care was taken to interview both decisionmakers as well as program implementers. The objective of the

TABLE AI-I: POPULATION ESTIMATES AND SAMPLE SIZE FROM PARTICIPATING CARIBBEAN COUNTRIES

Country	Population estimate[a]	Final sample	% of sample	Weighted % of sample
Antigua and Barbuda	64,000	2,158	13.7	1.5
Bahamas	279,000	1,787	11.4	5.6
Barbados	265,000	1,819	11.6	6.5
British Virgin Islands	19,000	400	2.5	0.4
Dominica	75,000	2,719	17.3	1.9
Grenada	99,000	1,255	8.0	2.4
Guyana	724,000	1,396	8.9	17.6
Jamaica	2,500,000	2,635	16.8	60.7
St. Lucia	145,000	1,526	9.7	3.5
Total	4,170,000	15,695	100	100

a. Population estimate from U.S. Department of Commerce websites for each country.

focus group was both triangulation (for the results) and to get the perspective of those who work with youth.

For the individual interviews, key informants with experience working with youth, or with strong knowledge regarding youth's reality, were selected. Specialized or specific informants from government institutions or NGOs, as well as specialists on specific areas, such as youth training and education, drugs, and sexuality, were selected.

The interviews were based on a structured interview guide. They lasted approximately one hour.

Qualitative Data Analysis

Using Pan American Health Organization (PAHO) survey data of school-going children in nine Caribbean Community (CARICOM) countries, the determinants of risky youth behavior were analyzed using parametric and nonparametric methodologies.

Data

The data are a cross-country, cross-sectional survey done in 1997–2000 by PAHO in collaborative with the ministries of health in the nine countries and the WHO Collaborating Center in Adolescent Health at the University of Minnesota, Minneapolis, Minnesota. All 19 CARICOM countries were invited to participate, and the following nine joined the regional survey: Antigua and Barbuda, the Bahamas, Barbados, the British Virgin Islands, Dominica, Grenada, Guyana, Jamaica, and St. Lucia. The final core survey contained 87 multiple choice questions dealing with school performance, school environment, alcohol and other drug use, sexual and reproductive history, physical and sexual abuse, moral behavior (honesty), violence, mental health and suicide, religiosity, family characteristics, relationships with others, general health, health care, and nutrition and body image.[1]

Data were collected in schools from 10- to 18-year-old children. Statisticians at the ministries of health carried out sampling procedures in each country. The sample size within each country was selected so that the sample was representative of school-going teenagers within each country and to ensure a power of 0.80 to detect differences among countries. The total sample included 15,695 students aged 10 to 18 (sample sizes and share of total population are given in table A1-1).

---

1. A draft questionnaire was reviewed by maternal and child health representatives from 19 Caribbean nations, then pilot tested on 105 young people. The instrument was revised, piloted again, and critiqued by more than 50 school-going young people.

It should be noted that these are not nationally representative samples of school-aged young people because they do not represent youth who leave school before graduating from secondary school. This imposes a bias in the data because, as shown by numerous studies, those who leave school and those who are absent on any given day (e.g., the day the survey was done) are at higher risk than their peers for nearly every negative outcome. Thus, what is presented by the data is the most positive picture, based on school-going youth. Approximately one-fifth (21.4 percent) were 16 to 18 years of age, 47.2 percent were 13 to 15, and nearly a third (31.4 percent) were aged 10 to 12. The difference in age distribution for males and females, although statistically significant, is not large enough to be of practical importance (<3 percent in each age category).[2]

Descriptive analyses were conducted for all variables of interest. Data on prevalence rates for each outcome are described as the proportion of students affected. Prevalence is reported by age group and by gender to better understand who is most affected within the sample. Rates are presented as proportions. Demographic subgroups were compared using standard bivariate tests such as chi-square statistics. Weighting was used in the analyses so that the results reflect the proportion of the population in each country. Although this approach gives more weight to some countries than others, it allows us to better describe the region as a whole. There were only 4 out of more than 200 possible responses for which weighted results were more than 5 percent different from unweighted results, suggesting that it is reasonable to present weighted results as representing the region and not solely the voice of larger countries. Table A1-2 shows that regression results by country are also very similar across countries, thus allowing us to generalize across the set of countries.

Data Analysis
Two methodologies are used to test the correlation between risk and protective factors and observed negative youth outcomes. First, logistic regression is used to estimate the correlation between having a risk or protective characteristic and the probability of engaging in risky behavior. A parameter estimate greater than one suggests a positive correlation between the behavior and the risk or protective factor, and a parameter estimate less than one suggests a negative correlation. We would have expected protective factors to carry coefficient estimates less than one, which would indicate that they are negatively correlated with the negative behavior, and risk factors with a coefficient estimate greater than one. Because there is a high correlation among the protective and risk factors, each regression includes only a single risk or protective factor and controls for gender and age group. The coefficient estimates presented in chapter 4 are significantly different from zero at the 1 percent level.

Five outcome (dependent) variables were used:

- perception of general health,
- ever had sexual intercourse,
- ever attempted suicide,
- violent behavior (a composite of four items, including if the respondent had carried a weapon to school in the past month and if he or she had been injured in a fight with a weapon), and
- problems due to alcohol and drugs (a composite of 10 questions, including the quantity of alcohol or drugs consumed in the previous week, whether ever had social problems due to substance use, whether ever engaged in risky behavior due to substance use, etc.).

---

2. Surveys with more than one-third of the items left blank were deleted from the sample. A total of 13 percent of the weighted sample was deleted for incompleteness. Surveys were also checked for invalid responses; only 2 percent of the sample was deleted for these reasons.

TABLE A1-2: FACTORS ASSOCIATED WITH RISK BEHAVIORS, BY RISK BEHAVIOR AND COUNTRY

Risky behavior	Risk or protective factor	Country 1	2	3	4	5	6	7	8	9
Ever had sex	Tries hard in school	1.01	0.64	0.68	0.84	0.81	0.91	0.78	0.82	0.93
	Connectedness to parent/family	0.67	0.50	0.92	0.43	0.54	0.61	0.57	0.54	0.38
	Attends religious services	0.91	0.90	0.93	0.81	0.85	0.87	0.83	0.87	0.79
	Sexual abuse	1.75	5.70	1.73	3.39	4.23	2.07	4.46	3.36	3.30
Ever attempted suicide	Tries hard in school	0.68	0.68	0.74	0.74	0.73	0.71	0.85	0.66	1.00
	Connectedness to parent/family	0.27	0.31	0.32	0.26	0.31	0.32	0.36	0.36	0.26
	Attends religious services	1.01	0.96	1.04	0.98	0.88	0.99	0.90	1.07	1.06
	Ever experienced any abuse	3.20	2.22	3.39	3.38	2.15	2.54	2.36	2.27	4.60
	Family member or friend attempted suicide	2.62	2.48	1.84	2.48	2.06	2.42	2.29	2.24	2.92
Ever involved in weapon-related violence	Tries hard in school	0.72	0.76	0.70	0.78	0.88	0.62	0.84	0.78	0.99
	Connectedness to parent/family	0.51	0.63	0.49	0.49	0.59	0.58	0.59	0.47	0.60
	Attends religious services	0.97	0.95	0.82	0.76	0.85	0.86	0.88	0.87	0.81
	Ever experienced any abuse	1.51	1.90	1.90	1.61	2.22	1.89	1.52	1.66	2.30
	Think about hurting or killing someone	2.45	3.02	3.67	4.35	3.42	2.83	2.63	3.31	5.45
	Parents have a problem with violence	2.64	1.51	2.39	2.62	3.50	3.57	1.98	1.65	2.60
Ever had problems due to alcohol or drugs	Tries hard in school	1.26	0.92	0.78	0.82	1.07	0.98	0.92	0.80	0.99
	Connectedness to parent/family	0.74	0.64	0.55	0.45	0.66	0.43	0.54	0.69	0.72
	Attends religious services	0.84	0.86	0.85	0.80	0.78	0.88	0.81	0.81	0.69
	Parent(s) has mental health problem	2.93	2.84	3.01	3.60	3.29	3.15	3.96	2.37	3.94
	Worried about substance abuse at home	2.67	1.98	3.31	3.58	4.42	4.24	2.94	3.64	2.19
	Parents have a problem with violence	2.19	2.79	3.66	4.57	2.41	3.61	3.03	3.34	5.66

Note: Odds ratios: >1 = risk; <1 = protective.

Source: PAHO Adolescent Health Survey (1999).

Nine predictor (independent) variables were used:

- how hard the person tries at schoolwork,
- attendance at religious services,
- thinks about hurting or killing someone,
- parents' problems with violence,
- parents with mental health problems,
- friend or family member who has committed suicide,
- parental and family connectedness (a composite variable of feeling that parents care, can tell parents about problems, other family members care, people in the family understand, family pays attention to the young person),
- victim of physical or sexual abuse, and
- parental substance abuse (alcohol or drugs).

The coefficient estimates show how well having a particular risk or protective factor explains the variance of the dependent variable, that is, how closely correlated they are. It does not show the magnitude of the effect or causality.

The second methodology uses nonparametric methods to identify the powerful effects of the presence of multiple protective or risk factors. The top three protective (or risk) factors were taken for each outcome. Selecting protective factor p_1, the likelihood of engaging in the risky behavior for youth with a high amount of p_1, but a low amount of characteristics p_2 and p_3, was measured. A similar exercise was done for p_2 and p_3. This exercise showed the marginal effects by protective factor. Next, the proportion of youth with various combinations of two of the three protective factors was calculated. Finally, the proportion of youth with all three protective factors and who engage in the risky behavior is calculated. A similar exercise was carried out for the risk factors.

Appendix 2

Lifetime Earnings from an Additional Level of Education for Select Countries by Sex

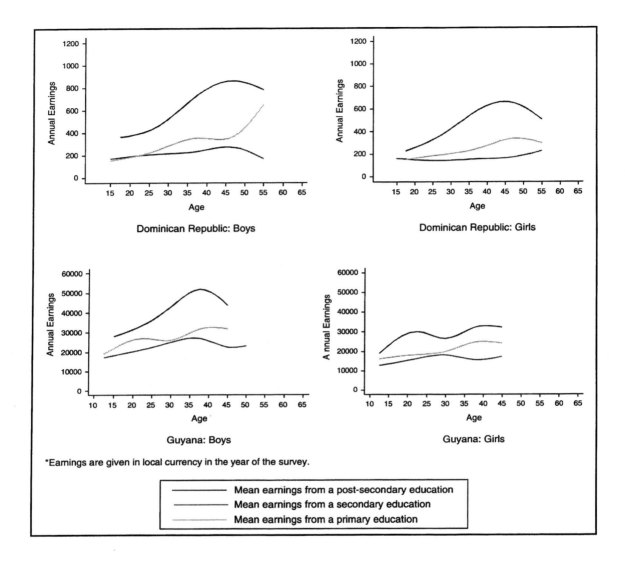

*Earnings are given in local currency in the year of the survey.

——————— Mean earnings from a post-secondary education
----------------- Mean earnings from a secondary education
··················· Mean earnings from a primary education

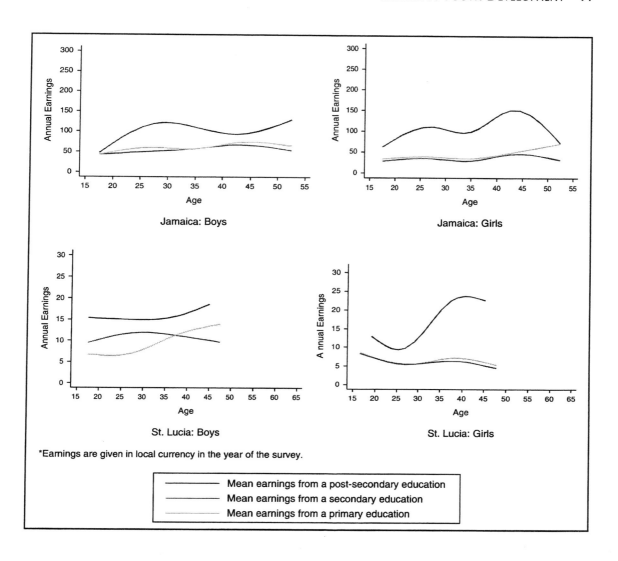

*Earnings are given in local currency in the year of the survey.

———————	Mean earnings from a post-secondary education
··················	Mean earnings from a secondary education
··················	Mean earnings from a primary education

Appendix 3

METHODOLOGY FOR COST CALCULATIONS, CHAPTER 5

Because of the scarcity of data in the Caribbean region, the methodology to estimate the costs in chapter 5 uses the country-specific numbers that could be obtained, but we also make bold assumptions that cost structures are similar across the Caribbean. These estimates can be further refined as additional data become available.

Crime and Violence

The costs of crime are difficult to estimate because of the scarcity of data on criminal activity and arrest, judicial, and incarceration rates and costs. However, enough data were available for five exercises that measure the financial social costs of youth criminal activity, the private social costs of youth criminal activity, the economic social costs of youth criminal activity, the increase in tourist receipts from a 1 percent decrease in youth crime, and the private social costs of youth criminal activity. Various calculations are carried out for Jamaica, St. Lucia, Trinidad and Tobago, and Barbados, depending on data availability.

Financial Social Costs of Youth Criminal Activity

The generation of this statistic requires the sum of two types of costs:

1. The product of the tangible costs of each crime type and the number of those crimes committed by youth that were reported in a country at that time was generated for each type of crime for which data were available. The sum across all crime types gives the total value of tangible crime costs annually.
2. The cost of arrest, prosecution, and (average) detention is multiplied by the number of youth crimes committed annually.

The exercise is carried out for Jamaica and St. Lucia, with the following assumptions:

- The victim compensation cost of the tangible costs by type of crime estimated in the United States (Roman and Farrell 2001) is a rough estimate of the tangible costs of these same crimes in St. Lucia and Jamaica, given in table 5-1 of the report.
- The tangible costs of possession of firearms (Jamaica) and drug offenses (Jamaica and St. Lucia) are zero.
- The cost of arrest, prosecution, and detention of an average criminal in Trinidad and Tobago approximates the costs in Jamaica and St. Lucia, and is equal to US$5,000 per crime (World Bank 1996).
- Youth crime data are given for Jamaica but not for St. Lucia. However, in Jamaica, approximately one-tenth of all crimes are prosecuted and 55 percent of all crimes are committed by youth so # crimes * (1/10) * (0.55) gives the total number of prosecuted youth criminals in St. Lucia. The annual prosecution of youth for each type of crime is as follows:

TABLE A3-1: ANNUAL PROSECUTION OF YOUTH

	St. Lucia	Jamaica
Number of youth convicted, by crime	4,140	1,266
Sexual assault	1.1%	2.8%
Murder and manslaughter	0.3%	2.34%
Grievous harm	16.0%	8.0%
Assaults	15.4%	—
Theft, robbery, larceny, extortion	35.2%	32.5%
Illegal firearms	—	7.6%
Dangerous drugs	7.7%	26.6%

Source: Data for St. Lucia are from ECLAC/CDCC (2001), and data for Jamaica are from Pantin (2000).

The costs missing from these calculations are the value of the property damage, expenditure on police force, and costs of *all* crimes, not just those that are prosecuted.

Private Social Costs

The cost of private security measures for Trinidad and Tobago ranges from US$5,036 to US$34,000 *per year*, of which US$3,969 are fixed costs and the remaining are annual recurrent costs. The fixed costs include installing security cameras, installing barriers to the house, or improving the safety of one's car, and the recurrent costs are primarily due to hiring a 24-hour guard. The total value of the security industry in the countries of study cannot be estimated, so we can only note that the figures generated omit this category, which will substantially underestimate the two costs. These values are derived from World Bank (1996).

Economic Social Costs

These costs are estimated for Jamaica and St. Lucia. The economic social costs are given by the sum of three components:

1. The forgone tax revenue of juveniles who are in prison: Assuming that those who are in prison would otherwise be employed or unemployed (not idle), the following equation is calculated for this component:

$$[\text{mean annual wage}/2 * 0.8 * (1\text{-male youth unemployment rate})] * 0.2$$

The mean annual wage is divided by 2 to account for the average six-month prison stay. The wage is multiplied by 0.8 to account for the lower wages of youth relative to adults. Finally, it is adjusted by the youth unemployment rate. The male wage and unemployment rates are used because most juvenile prisoners are men. A tax rate (income and consumption) of 20 percent is assumed.

2. The opportunity cost of resources used for prosecution, arrest, and detention: Assuming a return of 6 percent on an alternative use of investments, the total expenditures on prosecution, arrest, and detention (World Bank 1996) are multiplied by 0.06. This requires the assumption that the costs for Trinidad and Tobago approximate those in St. Lucia and Jamaica.

3. The opportunity cost of the tangible costs: Similarly, the total spent on tangible costs is multiplied by 0.06 to estimate the opportunity cost of the resources. The tangible costs are those outlined in table 5-1.

The Increase in Tourist Receipts from a 1 Percent Decrease in Youth Crime

To estimate the gain in tourist dollars due to a decrease in youth crime, we use the elasticities found in Levantis and Gani (2000), 1994 tourist flows and expenditures as reported by the Caribbean Tourism Organization, and 1994 crime rates as reported by the United Nations. A 1 percent decrease in youth crime was estimated to decrease the total crime rate by 6 percent. Applying the elasticity to this measure, total tourist flows were estimated to increase and, assuming that demand for tourist goods and services is perfectly elastic, the corresponding increase in tourist expenditures was generated. This was presented as a proportion of current tourist flows.

Private Economic Costs

Three components are estimated in this section:

1. Psychological costs of all crimes (cost to victim): Using the data from table 5-1 and applying the number of times the crime occurs from the above table, the intangible costs of crimes in Jamaica and St. Lucia are generated

2. Forgone benefits of resources spent on security (cost to victim): Similar to the opportunity cost of public expenditures, the total value of resources spent on security is multiplied by 0.06 to estimate the opportunity cost.

3. Forgone income of prisoner (cost to juvenile delinquent's family): The cost of forgone earnings is assumed to be equal to the youth annual wage (equal to 80 percent of the adult wage), discounted for the level of youth unemployment and multiplied by the average number of years of incarceration. In Trinidad and Tobago, the average prison stay was six months, so the same is assumed for St. Lucia and Jamaica.

The data sources used in these calculations are

- Direct cost of crime in terms of arrest, prosecution, and incarceration is US$5,000 per arrest (World Bank 1996)
- The number of youth and adult crimes convicted in Jamaica is from Pantin (2000)
- Mean wages were generated using the Jamaica labor force survey and the St. Lucia Living Standards Survey.
- The total number of crimes by country is given by the United Nations.
- The youth unemployment rate is from the International Labour Organisation

Adolescent Pregnancy

The costs of adolescent pregnancy reach far beyond the hospital cost of a young woman giving birth. Instead, they include all the additional costs over the lifetime of the adolescent mother and her child that are born privately or by society at large and that would not have occurred had the childbirth been postponed until the woman was 18 years old or older. The costs estimated for this exercise may be broken into six general areas, discussed below.

Mother's Forgone Annual Earnings and Tax Revenues

To measure the net loss to the mother's lifetime earnings that result from early school dropout and entry into less competitive or less lucrative jobs (in order to care for her child), the annual value of forgone earnings is given by

(mean adult earnings * adult unemployment rate – mean youth earnings
* youth unemployment rate) * (80/100)

where the first term is the net loss to the adolescent mother's earnings because she earns only a portion of the wage that she would have earned had she finished her education. This is multiplied by 0.8 to account for the gender wage gap that makes the net adult earnings rate an overestimate for women. Tax revenues are assumed to be 20 percent of income, whether collected through income or sales tax.

Annual Child Support

Adolescent mothers are shown to collect 32 percent less in child support from the childfathers than do nonadolescent mothers. The value of child support is approximately 18 percent of wages (Maynard 1996).[1] These private costs are born by society where

annual forgone child support = (annual wage * 0.18) – (annual wage * 0.18 * 0.32)

Government Income Transfers, Rent Subsidies, Food Stamps

Because young mothers will have lower earnings and less support from the childfathers, they will have a higher demand for public transfers than would other mothers. For several countries, the cost of these government benefits could not be measured. Given the scarcity of wide-reaching public assistance programs and the even rarer targeting of the programs toward young mothers (instead often targeting the elderly), an estimate of the value of government transfers that may be received by young mothers is derived from World Bank (1996). The following assumptions were made: For Jamaica, the weekly value of food stamps was assumed to be equal to one-half of the basic food basket adjusted for 11 percent of the population as recipients; for St. Lucia, no benefits were accrued to adolescent mothers because most benefits seem to reach one-person households (namely, the elderly); and for Trinidad and Tobago, the social benefits were assumed to accrue with equal probability to the whole population (World Bank 1996).

Medical Care

Adolescent mothers and their children require more health care than do older mothers and their children. The net additional cost is estimated to be 28.8 percent higher for the adolescent mother and her child than for the average citizen. Thus, the value used for the annual additional cost of medical care for the young mother and her child is 28.8 percent of the mean health care expenditure per person in each country.

Foster Care, Incarceration of Young Men, Productivity of Young Adults

Foster care programs are not well developed in the Caribbean region, so this was given a cost of zero. Crime costs were estimated as:

Cost of arrest, deterrence, and prosecution * probability of being arrested * Pr (commit a crime)

---

1. Child support is estimated to equal 18 percent of the average wage.

where the probability of being arrested is 4.3 percent (from the Jamaican data) and the probability of committing a crime is 25,000 per 1.5 million males (from the Jamaican data). Finally, the productivity of the child when he or she grows to adulthood is not included because it is difficult to put a price on a life.

Forgone Benefits of Alternative Use of Transfers and Health Costs

This is estimated by multiplying the net expenditures on transfers and health costs by 0.06, which is a healthy return to an investment. To generate the marginal cost of adolescent motherhood, the above cost components are summed according to their classification as given in the table below:

To estimate the lifetime costs, those costs that accrue to children (such as child support) are multiplied by 18 and those that accrue to the mother are multiplied by 50 (assuming that she lives until age 65, on average). The total is discounted at 6 percent.

The formulas used to generate table 5-4 are

Annual per birth—financial: financial health costs of mother and child + child support payments + government transfers + financial costs of crime

Annual per birth—economic: forgone tax revenue from mother + alternative use of government transfers and health expenditures

Annual per cohort—economic or financial: (annual per birth) * number of new adolescent mothers each year

Lifetime per cohort—economic or financial: [(annual child and mother costs per year while the child is dependent * 18) + (annual mother costs per year * (65-18-15))] *number of adolescent births in a cohort. A discount rate of 6% is applied to each term.

TABLE A3-2 CLASSIFICATION OF COST COMPONENTS OF ADOLESCENT MOTHERHOOD

	Financial costs	Economic costs
Private	▓ Health costs of mother and child	▓ Mother's forgone earnings ▓ Forgone consumption from not marrying ▓ Lower income and happiness of children who grow up poor, have health problems, have less education ▓ Social exclusion
Social	▓ Child support from the childfather ▓ Health costs of mother and child paid publicly ▓ Government transfers for aid to poor families, foster care ▓ Crime prevention, legal and justice system	▓ Forgone tax revenue from lower future income of mother ▓ Lower tax revenue from lower future income of child ▓ Forgone use of administrative resources for transfers and health care to adolescent mothers and their children ▓ Forgone benefits of alternative uses of health care and transfers to adolescent mothers and their children ▓ Economic costs of crime ▓ Loss to society of the marginal nonpecuniary contributions to society by the child and adolescent mother

HIV/AIDS

The cost to society of youth AIDS deaths and the deaths of those who contract HIV while young is measured as forgone earnings in this report. These would be the cost to society of not spending any money on drug regimens such as zidovudine (AZT) or HEART, instead relegating the individual to home care for the period of a year until death occurs (World Bank 2001b). Two measures are presented in chapter 5: (1) the cost to the country of AIDS deaths in the year 2000, the most recent year for which data on AIDS are available (PAHO); and (2) the total output forgone in the year 2000 due to *all* individuals who have died of AIDS since 1982, the first year for which PAHO provides data.

The following equation is used to generate the cost of forgone earnings attributable to AIDS deaths in the year 2000:

(# AIDS deaths ages 16–24 * mean annual wage * 0.8 * youth unemployment rate)
+ (# AIDS deaths ages 25–39 * mean annual wage * adult unemployment rate)

where the number of deaths for each age group is given by PAHO statistics on newly reported HIV/AIDS cases in 2000. The mean annual wage and youth and adult unemployment rates are derived from ILO statistics.

The assumptions in this calculation are

- The period between contraction of HIV and diagnosis of AIDS is 10 years.
- An individual with untreated AIDS dies within one year.
- The opportunity cost of the AIDS-related death is the total value of forgone income, which includes taxes paid. It underestimates the true cost because it does not consider AIDS orphans, psychological [costs, or other related negative externalities of the early death.
- The number of reported cases of HIV/AIDS is a proxy for the number of AIDS cases that develop per year. The number of HIV cases is unknown.
- A person with HIV is as productive as a healthy person; once HIV evolves into AIDS, the person's productivity falls to zero.
- No treatment.
- Youth earn 80 percent of adult mean wages.
- The wage elasticity of demand is zero.

To estimate the total losses in 2000 from all AIDS deaths of youth or of individuals who contracted HIV during their youth, the following is estimated:

(# AIDS deaths ages 16–24 in 2000 * mean annual wage * 0.8 * youth unemployment rate)
+ (#AIDS deaths ages 16–24 for 1982–1999 * mean annual wage * adult unemployment rate)
+ (#AIDS deaths ages 25–39 for 1982–2000 * mean annual wage * adult unemployment rate)

where the first term is the forgone earnings of youth who died of AIDS in 2000, the second term is the forgone adult earnings of youth who died of AIDS in previous years who are not contributing to productivity in 2000, and the third term is the value of forgone earnings attributable to all adult AIDS deaths since 1982 that are not contributing to gross domestic product (GDP) in 2000.

Unemployment

The unemployment section estimates the increase in GDP if youth unemployment were set equal to zero, equal to adult unemployment, or equal to youth unemployment in the United States.

The assumptions in this exercise are

- The wage elasticity of supply is set equal to 0 in the first column but equal to 2 in the second to estimates. The $\epsilon=2$ is derived from Arango and Maloney (2001), who generate wage elasticities for the manufacturing sector in Mexico and Argentina. The elasticities for youth in the Caribbean region are likely to be higher because they are primarily employed in services.

■ The unemployment rate is a random walk with a mean of 0. The year represented in the calculation for each country is assumed to be an average year. Because the years differ (based on the availability of unemployment data), world economic conditions will also differ

■ Real wages are constant. The wages are adjusted by the rate of inflation (CPI) to bring them to the year for which unemployment is measured.

■ Youth wages are 80 percent of adult wages because youth have less experience but higher levels of completed education.

■ Boys and girls earn the same real wages.

■ Women earn 80 percent of men's wages.

The relevant years of the unemployment rates used are shown in table A3-3.

■ Only those countries for which wages and unemployment rates were available are included in the sample. Wages were missing for Grenada, Dominica, Belize, St. Vincent and the Grenadines, and St. Kitts and Nevis.

■ Higher youth employment does not crowd out adult employment.

To calculate the percent increase in GDP due to a decrease of youth employment, the following equation was used:

{[(youth unemployment rate – target youth unemployment rate) * number of youth labor force participants] * [adult wage * 0.8]}/GDP

where the term in square brackets is the increased number of youth due to higher youth employment and the second term in square brackets is the youth wage. Multiplying these terms together is the total additional output due to productively employing more of the youth labor force. Finally, the total product is divided by the GDP to estimate the increase in GDP due to higher youth employment.

The exercise is repeated three times for girls and boys, where the target youth unemployment rate is set equal to:

1. *Zero:* This would be an ideal situation, though highly unrealistic. Thus, it should be interpreted as the upper bound of lost productivity.

TABLE A3-3: RELEVANT YEARS OF UNEMPLOYMENT RATE

Country	Survey Year
Antigua and Barbuda	1991
Barbados	1999
Dominican Republic	1996
Guyana	1992
Jamaica	1999
St. Lucia	1998
Suriname	1998
Trinidad and Tobago	1999

Source: ILO 1999.

2. *The adult unemployment rate:* This may be a feasible target if the productivity of the more educated young labor force rises to the level of the productivity associated with the higher productivity of adults. The demand elasticity of wages is set equal to –2 (Maloney and Arango 2003).

3. *The youth unemployment rate in the United States:* Given the high degree of migration to the United States, the two labor markets may move toward convergence. With perfect convergence, the youth unemployment rates should be equal. The demand elasticity of wages is set equal to –2.

The data are drawn from the following sources:

- wages: ILO adult wages,
- unemployment rate: ILO youth and adult unemployment rates,
- number of youth in the labor force: ILO,
- GDP: International Monetary Fund (IMF) international financial statistics reported in local currency, and
- inflation rate: IMF international financial statistics based on the CPI.

School Leaving

The measurement of net and total productivity loss due to early school leaving is a two-step process. First, an age earnings profile is constructed to measure the forgone earnings attributable to not completing an additional year of education. Using household and labor force surveys from Jamaica (1997), the Dominican Republic (1998), St. Lucia (1995), and Guyana (1999), average nonzero income by age group (in five-year intervals) and education group (by education level) are generated. The wages are multiplied by the probability of working at each age and education level to find an average wage per age and education group. These are used to construct age earnings profiles, which are the graphs of total earnings based on education level, given in appendix 2. Five-year intervals are used because the sample sizes are too small to robustly generate mean earnings per age group, and the education group is used because the surveys do not report grade level. The following assumptions are made:

- Earnings of a 60-year-old today are a proxy for real earnings of a 20-year-old today when he or she is 60 years old.
- Reported monthly wages are multiplied by 12 to estimate annual wages (Jamaica and Guyana), and weekly wages are multiplied by 4.3 and by 12 (St. Lucia).
- Wage earning begins at age 16 for primary and secondary school dropouts because the legal work age is 16 in most countries and work younger than age 16 is usually unpaid and in small businesses. Wage earnings begin at age 22 for postsecondary-educated individuals.
- Individuals are in the labor market until age group 45–55, depending on the country. The upper age is determined by data availability.
- The number of boys and girls who do not finish each grade level is equal. This is a bold assumption because girls have higher education rates than boys, especially in urban areas.
- The social rate of return is 6 percent.

This method is used rather than estimating a Mincer earnings equation and then using the estimates to plot the earnings path because that would constrain the returns to each level of education to be linear, which they clearly are not.

The forgone earnings from not completing the higher level of education are generated by summing the total lifetime earnings from education level E+1 and subtracting from it the total lifetime earnings from leaving school with education level E. The exercise is carried out for primary versus secondary education level and for secondary versus tertiary education and separately for men and women. These values are converted to U.S. dollars.

Finally, to calculate the lost productivity of *all* youth who were not in school in the observation year, the marginal rates are multiplied by the number of youth who were not in each level of school. Thus, the marginal gain from secondary education relative to primary education is multiplied by the percentage of students who did not enter secondary school and the marginal gain to postsecondary education relative to secondary education is multiplied by the number of secondary students who did not go on to postsecondary school. The number of students who did not enter each respective level of school is given in table A3-4.

The data are drawn from the following sources:

- Wages by age and education level: Jamaica Survey of Living Conditions (1997), Guyana Survey of Living Conditions (1999), National Survey of Income and Expenditure (Central Bank, Dominican Republic 1998), Living Standards Measurement Study for St Lucia (1995);
- Number of students who did not finish each grade level: World Development Indicators (World Bank, 1998–99); and
- Proportion of the employed labor force: household and labor market surveys.

TABLE A3-4: NUMBER OF STUDENTS WHO DID NOT FINISH THE RESPECTIVE GRADE LEVEL			
	Dominican Republic	**Guyana**	**Jamaica**
Primary	54,824	3,550	5,460
Secondary	267,453	21,007	22,526
Postsecondary	3,028,507	377,609	1,174,15

Source: World Development Indicators (World Bank 1998–99)

Appendix 4

CARIBBEAN YOUTH POLICIES AND PROGRAMS

TABLE A4-1: OVERVIEW OF NATIONAL YOUTH PROGRAMS, POLICIES AND LAWS RELATED TO YOUTH IN SELECT CARIBBEAN COUNTRIES

Country	Responsible Government Agency	Separate Youth Policy	Thematic Thrust	Services	Programmes/ Links to Other Programmes	Comments
Antigua and Barbuda	Youth Department, Ministry of Education, Youth, Sports and Community Development	No	Drugs, study skills, AIDS, career development, teen pregnancy, family and school relations, school leavers	✓ Junior achievement ✓ Peer counseling ✓ National summer camps ✓ Drug busters ✓ Continuing education		
The Bahamas	Youth Department, Ministry of Youth and Culture	Yes	Youth leadership, safe physical spaces, labor market preparation, citizenship, culture and history, literacy	✓ National youth research and resource center ✓ National media campaign ✓ Youth leadership training and organization, strengthening family ✓ Job readiness and enterprise scheme ✓ Personal development seminar ✓ Health, sports and recreation programme		
Barbados	Youth Affairs Division, Ministry of Education, Youth Affairs and Culture	No	Citizenship, culture, employment, nation building		✓ Youth Service ✓ Youth Development Programme ✓ Youth Entrepreneur Programme	Considered highly effective due to: political will and support; autonomous nature of the division; and effective information and research system.

Country	Policy	Lead Ministry/Department	Priority Areas	Youth Bodies/Programs	Comments
Belize	Yes	Ministry of Human Resources, Women's Affairs and Youth Development	Disaffected youth, gang violence and street crime	✓ National Youth Council	Effective processes to identify youth needs and tailor programs through cadre of youth officers working at the local and municipal levels.
Dominica	In draft	Ministry of Education, Sports and Youth Affairs	Drug prevention education		
Grenada	In draft	Ministry of Youth, Sports and Community Development		✓ National Youth Council of Grenada	Interest has not yet translated into effective programming. CYP currently advising on improving the organizational structure of the youth unit.
Guyana	Yes	Youth Department, Ministry of Labour, Human Services and Social Security	Leadership, anti sex discrimination, citizenship	✓ National Youth Council ✓ Youth Service Scheme ✓ Youth Employment Scheme	Hindered by size of the country and large geographical distribution of the population; weak public service structure affects overall effectiveness of public service (including youth).
Jamaica	Yes (currently under revision)	Youth Unit, Ministry of Education and Culture	Education and training, employment and empowerment strategies, health (including responsible parenting), drug abuse, recreation and leisure, values, attitudes and anti-social behavior, youth in community and nation building	✓ Special Training and Empowerment Programme (STEP) ✓ Human Employment and Resource Training (HEART) ✓ National Youth Service Programme ✓ National Youth Council	Effective at the national level due to the success of the National Center for Youth Development; weak at the field level; active NGO sector.

(continued)

TABLE A4-1: OVERVIEW OF NATIONAL YOUTH PROGRAMS, POLICIES AND LAWS RELATED TO YOUTH IN SELECT CARIBBEAN COUNTRIES (*CONTINUED*)

Country	Responsible Government Agency	Separate Youth Policy	Thematic Thrust	Services	Programmes/ Links to Other Programmes	Comments
St. Lucia	Department of Youth and Sports, Ministry of Education, Human Resource Development, Youth and Sports	Draft (approved by Cabinet)	Youth economic participation, youth education and training, crime prevention, substance abuse religious values, sports and recreation, culture, teen pregnancy, participation, health		National Youth Council	Considered to be highly effective due to long history of voluntary youth organizations (under the National Youth Council).
St. Vincent and Grenadines	Department of Youth, Ministry of Housing, Local Government and Community Development ?Ministry of Housing, Community Development, Youth and Sports	Draft	Group development and dynamics, leadership and communications, health and family life education, conflict resolution, peer counseling, parent education, drugs and alcohol abuse, small business development	Development education and training, outreach, communications and information, project support	✓ National Youth Commission ✓ National Commission for juveniles ✓ Youth Exchange	Continues to maintain a traditional welfare approach to youth rather than moving to youth development.

			Training and employment		
Trinidad & Tobago	Department of Youth, Ministry of Sport and Youth Affairs	Draft	District youth services, youth centers, youth placement service, youth resource and information service	✓ Youth Training and Employment Partnership Programme ✓ Apprenticeship Programme ✓ Apprenticeship for Industrial Mobilization ✓ Socially and Economically Disadvantaged Areas ✓ National Youth Council	Active NGO sector, of which SERVOL is exemplary; Public sector has a large staff but tend to be desk bound.

Source: Danns, Henry and LaFleur (1997); Youth of the United Nations; Country Profiles on the Situation of Youth; National Youth Policy (http://esa.un.org/socdev/unyin/comparea.asp)

*Sectors: education, labor, health, economy, justice, commerce/industry, culture/national affairs

TABLE A4-2: HUMAN RIGHTS INSTRUMENTS RATIFIED OR ACCEDED
RELATED TO THE RIGHTS OF YOUTH

Country	Number	Instruments Ratified or Acceded
Antigua and Barbuda	3	✓ Abolition of Slavery, the Slave Trade, and Institutions and Practices Similar to Slavery (UN/1956) ✓ Consent to Marriage, Minimum Age for Marriage and Registration of Marriages (UN 1962); ✓ Convention on the Minimum Age for Admission to Employment (ILO/1973).
Bahamas	1	✓ Convention on the Abolition of Slavery, the Slave Trade and Institutions and Practices Similar to Slavery (UN/1956)
Barbados	6	✓ Night Work of Young Persons: Industry (ILO/1948) ✓ Abolition of Slavery, the Slave Trade and Institutions and Practices Similar to Slavery (UN/1956) ✓ Discrimination in Education (UNESCO/1960) ✓ Consent to Marriage, Minimum Age for Marriage and Registration of Marriages (UN/1962) ✓ Civil and Political Rights (UN/1966) ✓ Economic, Social and Cultural Rights (UN/1966).
Belize	3	✓ Medical Examination of Young Persons: Sea (ILO/1921) ✓ Discrimination in Education (UNESCO/1960) ✓ Civil and Political Rights (UN/1966).
Dominica	6	✓ Medical Examination of Young Persons: Sea (ILO/1021) ✓ Abolition of Slavery, the Slave Trade, and Institutions and Practices Similar to Slavery (UN/1956) ✓ Discrimination in Education (UNESCO/1960) ✓ Civil and Political Rights (UN/1966); Economic, Social and Cultural Rights (UN/1966) ✓ Minimum Age for Admission to Employment (ILO/1973).
Dominican Republic	9	✓ Non-Industrial Occupations (ILO/1946) ✓ Night Work of Young Persons: Industry (ILO/1948) ✓ Abolition of Slavery, the Slave Trade and Institutions and Practices Similar to Slavery (UN/1956) ✓ Discrimination in Education (UNESCO/1960) ✓ Consent to Marriage, Minimum Age for Marriage and Registration of Marriages (UN/1962) ✓ Civil and Political Rights (UN/1966) ✓ Economic, Social and Cultural Rights (UN/1966)
Grenada	3	✓ Medical Examination of Young Persons: Sea (ILO/1921) ✓ Civil and Political Rights (UN/1966) ✓ Economic, Social and Cultural Rights (UN/1966)
Guyana	4	✓ Civil and Political Rights (UN/1966) ✓ Economic, Social and Cultural Rights (UN/1966) ✓ Minimum Age for Admission to Employment (ILO/1973) ✓ Vocational Guidance and Vocational Training: Human Resources Development (ILO/1975)

TABLE A4-2: HUMAN RIGHTS INSTRUMENTS RATIFIED OR ACCEDED RELATED TO THE RIGHTS OF YOUTH (CONTINUED)

Country	Number	Instruments Ratified or Acceded
Haiti	6	Medical Examination of Young Persons: Industry (ILO/1946); Medical Examination of Young Persons: Non-Industrial Occupations (ILO/1946); Night Work of Young Persons: Industry (ILO/1948); Suppression of the Traffic in Persons and of the Exploitation of the Prostitution of Others (UN/1949); and Abolition of Slavery, the Slave Trade and Institutions and Practices Similar to Slavery (UN/1956); and Civil and Political Rights (UN/1966).
Jamaica	4	Medical Examination of Young Persons: Sea (ILO/1921); Abolition of Slavery, the Slave Trade and Institutions and Practices Similar to Slavery (UN/1956); Civil and Political Rights (UN/1966) and Economic, Social and Cultural Rights (UN/1966).
St. Lucia	2	Medical Examination of Young Persons: Sea (ILO/1921); and Abolition of Slavery, the Slave Trade and Institutions and Practices Similar to Slavery (UN/1956).
St. Vincent and Grenadines	4	✓ Abolition of Slavery, the Slave Trade and Institutions and Practices Similar to Slavery (UN/1956) ✓ Discrimination in Education (UNESCO/1960) ✓ Civil and Political Rights (UN/1966) ✓ Economic, Social and Cultural Rights (UN/1966).
Surinam	3	✓ Abolition of Slavery, the Slave Trade and Institutions and Practices Similar to Slavery (UN/1956); ✓ Civil and Political Rights (UN/1966) ✓ Economic, Social and Cultural Rights (UN/1966)
Trinidad & Tobago	5	✓ Medical Examination of Young Persons: Sea (ILO/1921) ✓ Abolition of Slavery, the Slave Trade and Institutions and Practices Similar to Slavery (UN/1956) ✓ Consent to Marriage, Minimum Age for Marriage and Registration of Marriages (UN/1962) ✓ Civil and Political Rights (UN/1966) ✓ Economic, Social and Cultural Rights (UN/1966)

Source: Youth of the United Nations; Country Profiles on the Situation of Youth; Human Rights Instruments (http://esa.un.org/socdev/unyin/comparea.asp)

Table A4-3: Main Organizations Providing Services to Youth-At-Risk, St. Lucia

Name of Organization	Type of Organization	Target Group	Description Of Program
National Youth Council	NGO	Youth	Umbrella organization of 162 youth volunteer organizations from 18 braches in St. Lucia (17 community-based, one comprising student councils from around the island)
St. Lucia Crisis Center	NGO	Females (20–39 years)	Hotline, counseling and legal services for abused and battered women; public outreach program
Archdiocesan Youth Council	NGO	Catholic youth (nationwide)	Faith-based activities and retreats, retreats for youth
Center for Adolescent Rehabilitation and Education	NGO (Catholic Church)	Youth without a 2nd school placement	Five centers in both urban and rural areas; vocational courses as well as like skills, public speaking, rap sessions, and stress management
Junior Achievement	Private Sector	School-going youth	Teaches entrepreneurship, economic self-determination, business skills development; school-based program funded by Hewlett Packard; 1000 students trained in schools of which only 10–15 percent are male
Charterhouse High School and College of Continuing Education	Private	Youth who failed to get a 2nd school place	Secondary school preparation, self-esteem and self-employment training; affiliated with Institute of Counseling, which has a hot-line for abused and marginalized youth
Uptown Gardens' Schools Center	Public (quasi) (St. Lucia Women's Council)	Female youth (12–15 years)	Rehabilitation program for abused, neglected or abandoned girls who are on the verge of delinquency; services include counseling, career guidance, computer literacy, creative arts, language and technical skills training, family support and counseling, home management, physical fitness, job placement

TABLE A4-3: MAIN ORGANIZATIONS PROVIDING SERVICES TO YOUTH-AT-RISK, ST. LUCIA (CONTINUED)			
Name of Organization	**Type of Organization**	**Target Group**	**Description Of Program**
National Skills Training Center Inc.	Public (in cooperation with private sector)	Youth	Job training to assist youth make a transition to the working environment; training in agriculture, business, construction, crafts and furniture making, hospitality services and information technology; day care services available In collaboration with the Belfund,[1] provides access to start up capital for small businesses
Boys Training Center	Public	Males (12–16 years)	Home for underprivileged, delinquent boys who are referred through the juvenile court system; boys remain until their 18th birthday; services include training in basic numeracy, literacy skills and vocational subjects as well as social activities
Bureau of Health Education	Public (Ministry of Health)	Youth	Education and sensitization programs to reduce teen age pregnancy and deal with women's health issues.
Dept of Youth and Sports	Public	Youth (10–35 year olds)	Development of youth sporting facilities and initiatives to deal directly with youth issues
Drug Abuse Resistance Education	Public	Children and youth (5–12 years)	School based extension program to teach drug prevention; program promotes self-esteem, stress management, peer pressure management, self-motivation
Substance Abuse Secretariat	Public	Youth	Public awareness programs; formation of drug prevention clubs, and support workshops, seminars, and outreach programs

[1] Belfund, formally titled as the James Belgrave Memorial Fund has a focus on community development and youth development. It is an initiative of the Poverty Reduction Fund, which was established on the model of Social Investment funds in Latin America and The Caribbean with a broad holistic approach to poverty alleviation.

TABLE A4-4: SELECTED PUBLIC AGENCY/NGOS PROVIDING SERVICES TO YOUTH-AT-RISK, CARIBBEAN

Name of Organization	Type of Organization	Target Group	Description Of Program
National Youth Council, St. Vincent and the Grenadines*	NGO	Youth	Membership organization of 57 member youth associations and clubs founded in 1966, which provides income generation, sports, housing support, community development projects, and vocational training at the community level Supported by dues, fees and some limited governmental and international funding
Marion House, St. Vincent and the Grenadines*	NGO	Youth	Parenting education for teen parents; youth assistance for school drop-outs (vocational training in hairdressing, child care, sewing, etc); counseling, including substance abuse counseling; adult education; backyard gardening; interpersonal skills
Liberty Lodge, St. Vincent and the Grenadines*	NGO	Male youth (7–15 years)	Residential care, remedial education and vocational training (furniture making) for 25 youth (max. 2 year stay)
Youth Guidance Center, St. Vincent and the Grenadines*	Public (Ministry of Health)	Youth	Two Youth Guidance Centers (Barrouallie and Greggs Village) provide skills training for youth; Family life education in Owia
National Skills Training Programme, St. Vincent and the Grenadines*	Public	Unemployed youth (15–35 years)	Training for self-employment, 350 youth trained per year (65% female)
Youth Peer Education, Dominican Republic	NGO	Youth (16–19 years)	Train youth volunteers to be peer educators in sexual and reproductive health services for youth (with an emphasis on STIs and HIV prevention); 150 youth trained annually, 600 currently active; in 2000 peer educators worked with 6,879 direct beneficiaries and reached 48,641 indirect youth beneficiaries through presentations made
Youth Entrepreneurship Scheme, Barbados	Public (Division of Youth Affairs)	Youth (15–30 years)	Mentoring, training, technical and financial assistance to assist youth to start their own businesses

TABLE A4-4: SELECTED PUBLIC AGENCY/NGOs PROVIDING SERVICES TO YOUTH-AT-RISK, CARIBBEAN (CONTINUED)

Name of Organization	Type of Organization	Target Group	Description Of Program
Barbados Youth Service, Barbados	Public (Division of Youth Affairs)	Youth (16–22 years)	12-month training on self esteem, team building, academic training, including a 19 week job attachment program with private sector firms and public sector agencies

Source: Barker (1995)

TABLE A4-5: SELECTED NGOs PROVIDING SERVICES TO YOUTH-AT-RISK IN JAMAICA

Name of Organization	Target Group	Description Of Program
YMCA	Street Children	Academic program for street children and other programs
Children First	Street Children	
YWCA	Unemployed Girls	Operates school leavers institutes, skills training,
Women's Center	Teenage Mothers	Implemented through 7 main centers and 11 outreach centers island wide. Helps girls continue their education and/or referral for services and skills training
Rural Family Support Organization	Teenage mothers and young men	Provides academic and skills training, counseling and support in 3 rural parishes
Mel Nathan Institute	Youth 16 and over	Operates community college with skills training programs
Youth Opportunities Unlimited (YOU)	In-school youth	Mentoring program
Kingston Restoration Company—Necessary Education Training (NET)	Inner City youth between 10 and 16	Remedial education, arts and craft, computer studies, counseling and environment awareness and support to students not attending school for financial reasons.
Kingston Restoration Company—Youth Education Support System (YESS)	Students in the South side of Kingston	Seeks to develop leadership qualities through organized activities for high school students of the South Side of Kingston
St. Patrick's Foundation		Skills training, community gym and health clinic, community development workshops, remedial classes, CXC and GCE classes and job placement
Operation Friendship	Youth 16–23	Employment generation, education and training programs and primary health care, social work, day care services
Addiction Alert	Youth at-risk (including drug users)	Drug education and life skills programs offered in school One year rehabilitation and training for at-risk youth to become youth leaders, trainers and peer educators
Friends Hotline	Youth	Toll free telephone line that provides counseling and referral
Ashe	Youth	Provides training in the performing arts and remedial education to inner city youth.
Fathers Incorporated	Young men	Offers training workshops, conferences, counseling and micro enterprise development to help men develop positive image of fathering and to become better fathers
VOUCH	Adolescents	Health education and social services on behalf of children

Source: Blank (2000)

TABLE A4-6: JAMAICA PUBLIC PROGRAMS FOR YOUTH, FISCAL YEAR 1999/2000

Program	Responsible Ministry/ Agency	Description	Number Served	Total Program Budget (J$M)
HEART Academies	HEART/NTA	Skills training to out of school youth	9,900	643.8
Vocational Training Centers	HEART/NTA	Skills training to out of school youth	5,700	313.7
School Leavers Training Opportunities/ Apprenticeship	HEART/NTA	On-the-job training	5,100	67.4
Vocational Training Development Institutions	HEART/NTA	Training for technical vocational instructors	1,900	82.6
Community-Based Training	HEART/NTA	Community based training	8,500	395.3
Skills 2000	HEART/NTA, MOLSS, SDC	Community based training/ entrepreneurial development	2,200 (1998/99)	7.2 (1998/99)
National Youth Service	MOLGYCD	Work experience/ resocialization	1,600	98.4
LEAP	HEART/NTA, SDC	Remedial education, training and shelter for street children	230	27.0
Lift-Up Jamaica	UDC	Short term employment	3,700	1,300
Special Training and Empowerment Program	SDC	Training and community enterprise development	390	
Micro Enterprise Development Agency	MIDA	Microenterprise credit	8,000 (1998/99)	70.3
Jamaica Association of Adult Literacy (JAMAL)	MOEC	Literacy, numeracy training	11,600	
MICO Care Center	MOEC	Assessment and remediation for special learning needs	2,000	24.0
MICO Youth Counseling Research Development Ctr.	MOEC	Counseling for youth with behavioral/emotional problems	Unavailable	Not available
VOUCH		Health, education, social services	Unavailable	0.3
Sporting Programs	MOLSS	Sporting programs in schools and communities	215,200	Not available
Cultural Programs	MOEC/JCDC	Visual and performing arts programs	35,000–40,000	18.71
Family Services	MOH	Counseling, care and protection services	4,500	370.71
Abilities Foundation	MOLSS	Skills training for disabled	27 trainees	4.7
Police Youth Clubs	MONSJ	Sport, education and camps	22,160	
4 H Clubs	MOA	Education and training	64,300	40.7

Source: Blank (2000)

TABLE A4-7: TRINIDAD AND TOBAGO SKILLS TRAINING AND EMPLOYMENT PROGRAMS

Program	Age Range	Number of Centers	Training Duration	Skills Provided	Stipend/ [Fees]	Beneficiaries/ year	Expenditure
Youth Training and Employment Partnership Programme (YTEPP)	15–25	over 20 school-based and 5 full-time centers	6 months	numeracy, literacy, life skills, 70 skills courses in 14 occupational areas, preparation for micro-enterprise	None	10,000	TT$30m/year approx. TT$1,200/ student/cycle
Service Volunteer for All (SERVOL)				numeracy, literacy, life skills and attitudinal	[TT$5/month]	(1999 data)	approx. TT$4m/year
✓ Junior Life	16–19	10	—	development, skills		448	
✓ Adolescent Development		20	14 weeks	courses, technical training in computers		1,699	
✓ Skill-training	"	12	6 months	and electronics		1,672	
✓ Hi-Tech	"	3	3 months			384	
Youth Development and Apprenticeship Centers	14–21	5 (1 in Tobago; 1 for girls)*	2 years (residential) several months (trade centers)	preparation for exams, primary school leaving certificate, trades train-ing (agriculture, con-struction, domestic and commercial sector), job placement	$TT45/month; housing and meals	1,325 (250 girls; 750 boys, residential program) 325 (trade centers)	TT$17m/year approx. TT$15,000/ youth/year

Source: World Bank (2000)

TABLE A4-8: JAMAICA SAFETY NET PROGRAMS BENEFITING YOUTHS, 1998

Program	Ministry	Benefits to Youth	Annual Beneficiaries	Expenditures J$/US$ ('000,000)
School Feeding Program	Ministry Of Education And Culture	School lunch for students in selected secondary schools	302,000	J$395.2/US$10.8
School Fee Assistance	Ministry Of Education And Culture	Fee Assistance to students in selected secondary schools	38,500 (1997/98)	J$145.3/US$4.0
Grants to Tertiary Students	SLB	Grant to low income students enrolled in public universities	Unavailable	J$62.5/US$1.7
Student Welfare Programs	Ministry Of Education And Culture	Exam Fee Assistance to secondary and tertiary students	Unavailable	J$2.0/US$0.1
Food Stamps	Ministry of Labor and Social Security	Youth receive income support to extent that they are pregnant, have children under six or are indigent or incapacitated.	263,000	J$395.2/US$10.8
Outdoor Poor Relief	Ministry of Local Government, Youth and Community Development	Youth receive income support to extent that they live in poor families, have young children, and are indigent or incapacitated.	13,700	J$100.0/US$2.5
Economic and Social Assistance	Ministry of Labor and Social Security	Youth receive benefits to degree that they are incapacitated or have suffered natural or man-man disaster	23,200	J$121.0/US$3.3

Source: Blank, 2000

Program	Responsible Government Body	Eligibility Criteria for Benefits	Beneficiaries/ year	Annual[1] Expenditure
Self Help and Rehabilitative Efforts (SHARE)[2]	Ministry of Social and Community Development	▪ unemployed and no source of income ▪ not in receipt of other public assistance	6,800 households/ month (estimated 30,000 persons, including 20,000 children) (end-1997)	TT$3.5m
Unemployment Relief Program (URP)	Ministry of Local Government	▪ able-bodied unemployed between 17–65 ▪ no household income constraints	60,000 (Obs.: some youths may benefit directly)	TT$130
Public Assistance (PA)	Ministry of Social and Community Development	▪ female-headed household ▪ partners have deserted/ died or are incarcerated/ incapacitated ▪ certified disabled	48,620 (end-1997) (28,449 children)	TT$56m
School Feeding Program	Ministry of Education	▪ needy school children, informal targeting criteria	one-third of primary school population, app. 63,000 children	TT$80m
Civilian Conservation Corps (CCC)	Formerly, the Ministry of National Security, Defense Force Currently, YTEPP	▪ selection system prefers older candidates with low scores on several indices: education, level of employability, occupational status of household, and involvement in community activities ▪ age 18–25	5,891 (1997) 24,656 (1993–97)	TT$25m (1997)

TABLE A4-9: TRINIDAD AND TOBAGO SAFETY NET PROGRAMS BENEFITING YOUTHS

Source: World Bank (2000)
[1]Public expenditure;
[2]NGOs cooperate in program execution

TABLE A4-10: OVERVIEW OF YOUTH SERVING DONOR PROGRAMS IN THE CARIBBEAN

	HIV/AIDS	Health/ Family Life Education	Education	Health	Youth Empowerment	Economic/ Social Policy	Community Development	Urban Poverty/ Violence	Active In (Countries)
UNICEF	> Peer training in partnership with Red Cross[i] > Youth Information and support centers[ii] > Public information and advocacy[iii]	> Using classroom as the primary medium for transmission of messages > Empowering youth with knowledge and life skills (CARICOM countries)		Promotion of "youth-friendly" reproductive, physical, and emotional health services Trinidad and Tobago)	> Promotion of Youth participation > Capacity building of National Youth Councils (St. Vincent and the Grenadines, Dominica) > Promotion of national youth policies (Dominica, St. Kitts and Nevis) > Jamaica: Youth Information Centers at the heart of the Adolescent development and Participation program > Support CARICOM youth programmes	> Promotion of "youth-friendly" policies	> Youth and community empowerment		English and Dutch speaking Caribbean* (Coordinated from Barbados Office); Jamaica; Cuba; DR; Haiti; Guyana, Suriname

EU			> Technical and vocational training > Education sector reform > Education infrastructure > Institutional strengthening of Community Colleges	> Drug programs > Health infrastructure	> Social Investment Funds (Mainstreaming approach)	> Social Investment Funds	Jamaica, St. Kitts, St. Vincent, Barbados, Dominica, St. Lucia, Antigua. Regional Program.
DFID			> Education reform (access and quality of post-primary education) (mainstreaming of youth issues)	>Drug eradication		>Urban poverty and violence project / Inner cities renewal project (Jamaica)	British Overseas Territories, Caribbean regional Program, Jamaica. Cuba, DR, Guyana
PAHO	HIV/AIDS program	Health/family education	>Tobacco use program >Mental health promotion >Adolescent Health Surveys in nine (9) countries				Bahamas[iv], CPC Barbados[v], Cuba, DR, Guyana, Surinam, Haiti, Trinidad and Tobago, Jamaica[vi]

(continued)

TABLE A4-10: OVERVIEW OF YOUTH SERVING DONOR PROGRAMS IN THE CARIBBEAN (CONTINUED)

	HIV/AIDS	Health/Family Life Education	Education	Health	Youth Empowerment	Economic/Social Policy	Community Development	Urban Poverty/Violence	Active In (Countries)
CIDA	> Expanded support in the Caribbean (ESAC) Assistance to CAREC HIV/AIDS Program	> Gender Equality Program Responsive Grant Funding (gender socialization in schools, non-violent parenting skills for single/young parents	> Sub-regional education sector reform for primary and secondary schools; learning resources; learning outcomes for IT, math and science; training systems for school managers; curriculum development		> CFLI small grants program (Canada Fund for local initiatives) > Judicial and legal reforms in the OECS > Caribbean Regional Human Resource Development Program for Economic Competitiveness (CPEC) (skills training and re-tooling in major sectors)	> CFLI small grants program > OECS Micro and Small Enterprise Development Project		>Small grants program	All OECS countries including Anguilla and BVI; CPEC Project also covers Guyana, Jamaica, Belize and Suriname.
Commonwealth Youth Programme					> strengthening youth ministries > youth participation > Human Resource Development	> Economic enfranchisement program > Youth credit initiative > Human Resource Development			English Commonwealth countries

					Countries
UNFPA	Strengthening Adolescent Sexual Health programs	Improve access for youths through: > Reproductive health Program > Family Planning			21 English and Dutch speaking countries* Cuba Dominican Republic Haiti
UNDP	Reform of class-room culture	> Entrepre-neurship; > information technology > Social Policy Development	Attention to youth in com-munity develop-ment	S	Barbados (plus 10 Organization of Eastern Caribbean States)**; Cuba; DR; Jamaica; T and T; Suriname; Netherlands Antilles.
USAID	Adolescent reproductive health, youth-friendly clini-cal services; work through peer mes-sages, mass media, edu-cation etc	> 'Uplifting Adolescents' program includes community-based life skills program > Parenting program	Remedial read-ing and math for drop-outs and students doing poorly		Caribbean Regional pro-gram (emphasis on OECS**) Dominican Republic, Haiti, Guyana, Jamaica

*Anguilla, Antigua and Barbuda, Aruba, the Bahamas, Barbados, Bermuda, British Virgin Islands, Cayman Islands, Dominica, Grenada, Guyana, Jamaica, Montserrat, Netherlands Antilles, St. Kitts and Nevis, St. Lucia, St. Vincent and the Grenadines, Suriname, Trinidad and Tobago, Turks and Caicos.

**Antigua and Barbuda, Anguilla, Barbados, British Virgin Islands, Dominica, Grenada, Montserrat, St. Kitts and Nevis, St. Lucia, St. Vincent and the Grenadines.

[i] Dominica, BVI, Grenada, St. Lucia, Barbados, Montserrat.

[ii] Barbados, St. Lucia, St. Vincent and the Grenadines, Dominica, Trinidad and Tobago.

[iii] St. Kitts and Nevis, St. Lucia, Barbados, Suriname, Antigua and Barbuda, St. Vincent and the Grenadines, Grenada.

[iv] Also serves Turks and Caicos

[v] Also serves Anguilla, Antigua and Barbuda, British Virgin Islands, Dominica, French Guiana, Grenada, Guadeloupe, Martinique, Montserrat, and Saint Bartholomew, Saint Kitts and Nevis, Saint Lucia, Saint Martin, Saint Vincent and the Grenadines

[vi] Also serves Bermuda and Cayman Islands.

BIBLIOGRAPHY

Alexis, A. 2000. "Mainstreaming Youth in the Development Process." Public Lecture to Mark Youth Month 2000, University of Technology, Jamaica." Commonwealth Youth Programme, Guyana Processed.

Ayres, R. 1998. *Crime and Violence as Development Issues in Latin America and the Caribbean.* Washington, D.C.: World Bank.

Barker, G. 1995. "Situational Analysis of Drug Abuse among Youth At-Risk in the Caribbean: A Needs Assessment of Out-of-School Youth in St. Vincent and the Grenadines, Trinidad and Tobago, St. Maarten and Jamaica." UNDCP.

———. 1996. "Integrated Service Models For Youth: An Analysis of Selected International Experiences." World Bank, Washington, D.C. Processed.

———. 1998. "Boys in the Hood, Boys in the Bairro: Exploratory Research on Masculinity, Fatherhood and Attitudes toward Women among Low Income Young Men in Chicago, USA, and Rio de Janeiro, Brazil." Paper presented at the IUSSP/CENEP Seminar on Men, Family Formation and Reproduction, May 13–15. Buenos Aires.

Barker, G., and M. Fontes. 1996. "Review and Analysis of International Experience with Programs Targeted on Youth At-Risk." LASHC Paper Series 5. World Bank, Washington, D.C.

Barriteau, E. 2001. *The Political Economy of Gender in the Twentieth-Century Caribbean.* New York: Palgrove.

Barrow, C. 2001. *Children's Rights, Caribbean Realities.* Kingston: Ian Randle.

Benson, P. 1997. *All Kids Are Our Kids.* San Francisco: Jossey-Bass.

Blank, Lorraine. 2000. "Youth At-Risk in Jamaica Note." World Bank, Washington, D.C. Processed.

Blum, Robert. 2002. "Adolescent Health in the Caribbean." Draft. LCSPG/World Bank, Washington, D.C.

Blum, R. W. 1998. "Healthy Youth Development as a Model for Youth Health Promotion: A Review." *Journal of Adolescent Health* 22(5):368–75.

Blum, R., and P. Rinehart. 1997. *Reducing the Risk: Connections that Make a Difference in the Lives of Youth*. Minneapolis: Division of General Pediatrics and Adolescent Health, University of Minnesota.

Blum, R., T. Beuhring, M. L. Shew, L. H. Bearinger, R. E. Sieving, and M. Resnick. 2000. "The Effects of Race, Income and Family on Adolescent Risk-Taking Behaviors." *American Journal of Public Health* 90(12):1879–84.

Burton L. M., K. W. Allison, and D. Obeidallah. 1995. "Social Context and Adolescence: Perspective on Development among Inner-City African-American Teens." In L. C. Crockett and A. C. Crouter, eds., *Pathways through Adolescence*. Hillsdale, N.J.: Erlbaum.

Buvinic, M., and A. Morrison. 2001. "Violence Control." Technical Notes: Violence Prevention, Technical Note 6. Inter-American Development Bank, Washington, D.C.ehttp://www.iadb.org/sds/soc/publication/publication_546_1291_e.htm.

CAREC member countries. 2000. "Quarterly AIDS Surveillance Reports Submitted to CAREC's Epidemiology Division." Port Of Spain.

Coleman, J. 1988. "Social Capital in the Creation of Human Capital." *American Journal of Sociology* 94(suppl):95–120.

Danns, G. K., B. I. Henry, and P. LaFleur. 1997. *Tomorrow's Adults. A Situational Analysis of Youth in the Commonwealth Caribbean*. London: Commonwealth Secretariat.

Deosaran, R. 1992. *Social Psychology in the Caribbean*. Trinidad: Longman.

Eckstein, Zvi, and Kenneth Wolpin. 1999. "Why Youths Drop out of High School: The Impact of Preferences, Opportunities, and Abilities." *Econometrica* 67(6):1295–1339.

ECLAC/CDCC. 2001. "Developing Social Policy for Youth with Special Reference to Young Men in St. Lucia." Draft. Castries, St. Lucia.

Feldman, S., and G. Elliott. 1997. *At the Threshold: The Developing Adolescent*. Cambridge, Mass.: Harvard University Press.

Ferber, T., and K. Pittman. (with T. Marshall). 2002. *Helping All Youth to Grow Up Fully Prepared and Fully Engaged*. Washington, D.C.: The Forum for Youth Investment.

Furstenberg, F., and M. Hughes. 1995. "Social Capital and Successful Development among At-Risk Youth." *Journal of Marriage and the Family* 57:580–92.

Gacitúa, E., C. Soto, and S. H. Davis. 2001. *Social Exclusion and Poverty Reduction in Latin America and the Caribbean*. San José, Costa Rica: FLACSO/World Bank.

Garmezy, N. 1985. "Stress Resistant Children: The Search for Protective Factors." In J. E. Stevenson, ed., *Recent Research in Developmental Psychopathology*, supplement 4:213–33 of the *Journal of Child Psychology and Psychiatry and Allied Disciplines*. Oxford: Pergamon Press.

———. 1991. "Resiliency and Vulnerability to Adverse Developmental Outcomes Associated with Poverty." *American Behavioral Scientist* 34:416–30.

Green, C. 1994. "Historical and Contemporary Restructuring and Women in Production in the Caribbean." In H. Watson, ed., *The Caribbean in the Global Political Economy*. Boulder and London: Lynne Rienner.

Greenwood, P. W., K. E. Model, C. P. Rydell, and J. Chiesa. 1996. *Diverting Children from a Life of Crime: Measuring Costs and Benefits*. Santa Monica, Calif.: Rand Corporation.

Hahn, A. 2002. "Does America Have a Youth Development Policy?" *Youth & Policy, the Journal of Critical Analysis* 76:66–76.

Haveman, R., and B. Wolfe. 1984. "Schooling and Economic Well-Being: The Role of the Non-Market Effects." *Journal of Human Resources* 19:377–407.

Huggins, G. 1998. *Youth in Caribbean Development*.

International Labour Office (ILO). 1999. *Decent Work and Protection for All: Priority of the Americas*. Report of the Director-General. Fourteenth Regional Meeting of ILO American Member States, August 1999. Lima, Perú. Geneva: ILO.

James, D. W., ed. 1997. *Some Things DO Make a Difference for Youth: A Compendium of Evaluations of Youth Programs and Practices*. Washington, D.C.: American Youth Policy Forum.

James, D. W., ed. (with S. Jurich). 1999. *MORE Things That DO Make a Difference for Youth: A Compendium of Evaluations of Youth Programs and Practices, Volume II*. Washington, D.C.: American Youth Policy Forum.

James-Bryant, M. 1992. "Challenges Facing Caribbean Youth as the Region Approaches the 21st Century: Survival or Destruction." Submission to the West Indian Commission.

Le Franc, E. 2001. "Child Abuse in the Caribbean. Addressing the Rights of the Child." In C. Barrow, ed., *Children's Rights, Caribbean Realities*. Kingston: Ian Randle.

Levantis, Theodore, and Azmat Gani. 2000. "Tourism Demand and the Nuisance of Crime." *International Journal of Social Economics* 27:959–67.

Lewis, L. 1995. "The Social Reproduction of Youth in the Caribbean." In L. Lewis and R. C. Carter, eds., *Essays on Youth in the Caribbean*. Cave Hill, Barbados: Institute of Social and Economic Research, University of the West Indies.

———. forthcoming. "Caribbean Masculinity at the Dawn of the New Millenium." In R. Reddock, ed., *Interrogating Caribbean Masculinity*. Port of Spain: University of the West Indies Press.

Luther, David, Arlette St. Ville, and Julia Hasbún. 2002. "Caribbean Qualitative Youth Study: Dominican Republic and St. Lucia" Draft. LCSPG/World Bank, Washington, D.C.

Maloney, W. and P. Fajnzylber. 2003. "Comparing Consistent Dynamic Estimates of Labour Demand Relations Across Countries: What can we learn?" Universidade Federal de Minas Gerais, Belo Horizonte, Brazil.

Masten, A. S., and M. G. J. Reed. 2000. "Resilience in Development." In C. R. Snyder and S. J. Lopez, eds., *Handbook of Positive Psychology*. New York: Oxford University Press, 2002.

Maynard, Rebecca 1996. "The Cost of Adolescent Childbearing." In R. Maynard, ed., *Kids Having Kids*. Washington, D.C.: Urban Institute.

McAlister, A. 1998. *Juvenile Violence in the Americas: Innovative Studies in Research, Diagnosis and Prevention*. Washington, D.C.: PAHO.

McNeely, C. A., M. L. Shew, T. Beuhring, R. Sieving, B. C. Miller, and R. W. Blum. 2002. "Mother's Influence on Adolescents' Sexual Debut." *Journal of Adolescent Health*, Sept 31: 3: 256–265.

Meeks-Gardener, J. 2001. "A Case Control Study of Family and School Determinants of Aggression in Jamaican Children." PIOJ Policy Department Unit Sixth Working Paper. PIOJ, Kingston.

Miller, E. 1999. "Commonwealth Caribbean Education: An Assessment." In E. Miller, ed., *Educational Reform in the Commonwealth Caribbean*. Washington D.C.: Inter-American Agency for Cooperation and Development.

Miller, E., D. Jules, and L. Thomas. 2000. *Pillars for Partnership and Progress. The OECS Education Reform Strategy: 2010*. Castries, St. Lucia: OECS.

Morales, C. 2001. "Youth and Social Exclusion in Chile." In E. Gacitúa Soto and S. Davis, eds., *Social Exclusion and Poverty Reduction in Latin America and the Caribbean*. San José, Costa Rica: FLACSO/World Bank.

Neild, W. 2001. "The Role of Police in Violence Prevention." Technical Notes: Violence Prevention, Technical Note 9. Inter-American Development Bank, Washington, D.C. http://www.iadb.org/sds/soc/publication/publication_546_1291_e.htm.

Pantin, D. 2000. *Revisiting the Challenge of Youth Employment in the Caribbean*. Trinidad and Tobago: ILO.

Patterson, J., and R. W. Blum. 1996. "Risk and Resilience among Children and Youth with Disabilities." *Archives of Pediatric and Adolescent Medicine* 150:692–98.

Patterson, O. 1975. *The Sociology of Slavery: An Analysis of the Origins, Development and Structure of Negro Slave Society in Jamaica*. London: Farleigh Dickenson University Press.

Planning Institute of Jamaica (PIOJ). 1999. *Economic and Social Survey of Jamaica*. Kingston: PIOJ.

Rees, Daniel, Laura Argys, and Susan Averett. 2001. "New Evidence on the Relationship between Substance Use and Adolescent Sexual Behavior." *Journal of Health Economics* 20:835–45.

Resnick, M. and Mohammedreza Hojat. 1998. "Protecting Adolescents from Harm: Findings from the National Longitudinal Study on Adolescent Health." *Journal of the American Medical Association* 278(10):823–32.

Rock, L. 2001. "Child Abuse in Barbados." In C. Barrow, ed., *Children's Rights, Caribbean Realities*. Kingston: Ian Randle.

Rodríguez, E. 2000. *Políticas públicas de juventud en República Dominicana: Perspectivas y desafíos para el periodo 2001–2004*. Santo Domingo: Organización Iberoamericana de Juventud.

Roman, John, and Graham Farrell. 2001. "Cost-Benefit Analysis and Crime Prevention." Draft. Urban Institute, Washington, DC.

Roth, J, J. Brooks-Gunn, L. Murray, and W. Foster. 1998. "Promotion of Healthy Adolescents: Synthesis of Youth Development Program Evaluations." *Journal of Research on Adolescence* 8(4):423–59.

Russell-Brown, P., P. Engle, and J. Townsend. 1994. *The Effects of Early Childbearing on Women's Status in Barbados*. Washington, D.C.: International Center for Research on Women.

Rutter, M. 1993. "Resilience: Some Conceptual Considerations." *Journal of Adolescent Health* 14:626–31.

Safa, H. 1994. *The Myth of the Male Breadwinner: Women and Industrialization in the Caribbean*. Boulder, Colo.: Westview Press.

Samms-Vaughan, M. 2001. "The Caribbean Child's Right to Education. Educational Provision, Socio-economic and Family Factors and School Achievement." In C. Barrow, ed., *Children's Rights, Caribbean Realities*. Kingston: Ian Randle.

Singh, W. 2001. "Children, the Law and Juvenile Justice." In C. Barrow, ed., *Children's Rights Caribbean Realities*. Kingston: Ian Randle.

Suárez, E., and C. Quesada. 1999. "Communication as a Tool for Social Change." In A. Morrison and Loreto Biehl, eds., *Too Close to Home. Domestic Violence in the Americas*. Washington, D.C.: Inter-American Development Bank.

Tejada Holguin, R., J. Herold and L. Morris. 1992. *Republica Dominica Encuesta Nacional de Jóvenes, 1992*. Instituto de Estudios de Población y Desarrollo (Centre for Disease Control and Prevention).

Trouillot, M. 2001. "Social Exclusion in the Caribbean." In E. Gacitúa Soto and S. Davis, eds., *Social Exclusion and Poverty Reduction in Latin America and the Caribbean*. San José, Costa Rica: FLACSO/World Bank.

UNDCP. 1997. *Economic and Social Consequences of Drug Abuse and Illegal Trafficking*. UNDCP Technical Series 6. New York: United Nations.

UNICEF. 2002. "Social Initiatives at the Community Level in Support of Youth and Adolescent Development. Integrated Community Models for a Healthy Start and Safe Passage to Adulthood." Paper presented at the Eighth Annual Retreat of the International Development Partners (IDPs) in Jamaica, November 13–15. Runaway Bay, Jamaica.

Werner, E., and R. Smith. 1982. *Vulnerable but Invincible*. New York: McGraw-Hill.

West Indian Commission. 1992. *Time for Action*. Kingston: University of the West Indies Press.

Williams, L. 2001. "Anywhere yuh be, yuh not safe: adolescence and violence in Jamaica." Final draft for UNICEF and UNFPA, September 2001. Kingston, Jamaica.

Williams, L. 2002. "A Review of the Issues Arising from Selected Quantitative and Qualitative Literature on Youth in the Caribbean." Draft. LCSPG/World Bank, Washington, D.C.

Williams, S. 2001. " 'The Mighty Influence of Long Custom and Practice': Sexual Exploitation of Children for Cash and Goods in Jamaica." In C. Barrow, ed., *Children's Rights, Caribbean Realities*. Kingston: Ian Randle.

World Bank. 1996. *Poverty Reduction and Human Resource Development in the Caribbean*. Washington, D.C.: World Bank.

World Bank. 1999. *Consultations with the Poor.* Washington, D.C.: World Bank.

————. 2000a. *HIV/AIDS in the Caribbean: Issues and Options.* Washington, D.C.: World Bank.

————. 2000b. "Trinidad and Tobago. Youth and Social Development. An Integrated Approach for Social Inclusion." Report 20088-TR. World Bank, Washington, D.C.

————. 2001a. *Dominican Republic Poverty Assessment.* Washington, D.C: World Bank.

————. 2001b. "A Review of Gender Issues in the Dominican Republic, Haiti and Jamaica." Report 21866-LAC. World Bank, Washington, D.C.

————. 2002. *Optimizing the Allocation of Resources among HIV Prevention Interventions in Honduras.* Washington, D.C.: World Bank.

Wyatt, G. E., E. Le Franc, M. B. Tucker, B. Bain, B. Mitchell-Kernan, and D. Simeon. 1993. "Sexual Decision Making among Jamaicans: Final Report." Submitted to Family Health International.